What experts and the media ~~~~~~~ core concepts of *The Buffer Zone Diet*

"Intentional eating with mindful attention to the timing and frequency of eating occasions could lead to healthier lifestyle and cardiometabolic risk-factor management."

— AMERICAN HEART ASSOCIATION

"The discovery of *The Buffer Zone Diet* is a significant achievement and contribution to the field of weight management, and it will be your last stop on your path to weight loss and good health."

— DR. NINA, AUTHOR OF *FOOD FOR THOUGHT*

"Eating well isn't just about what you eat, say heart experts, but when you eat."

— *TIME* MAGAZINE

"What you eat makes a difference. Just counting calories won't matter unless you look at the kinds of calories you're eating."

— DR. DARIUSH MOZAFFARIAN, CARDIOLOGIST & EPIDEMIOLOGIST AT HARVARD SCHOOL OF PUBLIC HEALTH

"Meal timing, frequency may play role in preventing heart disease."

— CBS NEWS

"The American diet is said to be increasingly energy-rich but nutrient poor. To help improve the nutrient-to-energy ratio, the Dietary Guidelines for Americans recommend that consumers replace some foods in their diets with more nutrient-dense options."

— ADAM DREWNOWSKI

"Eat 'mindfully' rather than mindlessly."

— *FORBES*

"The amount (weight or volume) of food consumed affects the satiating potency of a food, independent of its energy content."

– The American Journal of Clinical Nutrition

"When and how often you eat may cut the risk of obesity and heart disease."

– ABC World News Tonight

"Blast fat, lower your cholesterol, and reduce inflammation. You can do it while you're asleep! Learn how shifting the times you eat can help reset your body."

– Dr. Oz

"When you eat can be as important as what you eat."

– NBC's Today

"Meal timing may affect health due to its impact on the body's internal clock."

– Huffington Post

"In the same way that I tell my patients 'I'd rather you do three repetitions the right way than five repetitions the wrong way', the goal of *The Buffer Zone* is maximizing your experience to get optimal results for nurturing and fueling your body."

– Vivian Eisenstadt, MPT CPT
a.k.a. The Brooklyn Healer

"Exercise well for your heart but eat well for your weight."

– Dr. Lara Dugas

"Of all the books about diets out there, *The Buffer Zone* is the only one I put in the hands of all of my friends, clients, and patients."

– Dr. John Philip Nesic, MD LSA RE

The **BUFFER ZONE**™ Diet

IT'S NOT JUST *WHAT* YOU EAT, IT'S *WHEN* YOU EAT.
HARNESS YOUR HIDDEN FUEL FOR A SLIMMER AND HEALTHIER YOU.

FRED CUELLAR

"Not everything that counts can be counted,
and not everything that can be counted counts"
— WILLIAM BRUCE CAMERON

MaxVera Publishing

The Buffer Zone Diet: It's Not Just What You Eat, It's When You Eat. Harness Your Hidden Fuel for a Slimmer and Healthier You

For information about this title or to order other books and/or electronic media, contact the publisher:
MaxVera Publishing
4265 San Felipe Ste. 960 Houston TX 77027
713-622-0830
www.maxverapublishing.com
mv@maxverapublishing.com

Library of Congress Control Number: 2017905641

ISBN: 978-0-9989091-0-3 (Hardcover)
        978-0-9989091-1-0 (Softcover)
        978-0-9989091-2-7 (eBook)

Printed in the United States of America

Cover and Interior design: 1106 Design

Publisher's Cataloging-in-Publication
(Provided by Quality Books, Inc.)

Cuellar, Fred, author.
    The buffer zone diet : how to harness your hidden
fuel for a slimmer and healthier you / Fred Cuellar.
        pages cm
        Includes bibliographical references.
        ISBN 978-0-9989091-0-3
        ISBN 978-0-9989091-1-0
        ISBN 978-0-9989091-2-7

    1. Reducing diets.   I. Title.

RM222.2.C7787 2017   613.2'5
                                  QBI17-753

Disclaimer: We urge our readers to seek medical or professional advice before beginning any weight-loss program, exercise, training regime, or any diet or meal plan.

To Britta,
All the Best

Acknowledgement

I n 1927, Hermann Hesse wrote the novel entitled *Siddhartha*. His book deals with the personal journey of a man named Siddhartha on his road to self-discovery.

In Hesse's masterpiece, that would later receive the Nobel Prize in Literature in 1942, he takes us on the same life journey as Siddhartha as he begins to unfold the meaning of life.

At one point in the story, our hero comes face-to-face with a wealthy man and asks him if he can teach him how to be wealthy, to which the wealthy man said (and I'm paraphrasing here), "I didn't become a rich man by giving things away. What can a man with no possessions possibly have to offer me?" Siddhartha answered, "I can think, wait, and fast."

The wealthy man appeared puzzled (as most of us would be). But with those three words Siddhartha opened the doors to the universe.

The key is our ability to weigh options and see that everything is a reflection of us, the ability to be patient and wait for what you truly want instead of settling, and the ability to tame the beast of hunger so that it serves you versus you serving it. Siddhartha is Sanskrit for Siddha, which means "achieved" and Artha, which means "what is searched for".

For all these things I am grateful, and for all these things I dedicate this book to all the Siddharthas out there searching for their truth.

Table of Contents

Foreword
By Dr. Nina

"'ve lost the same twenty pounds over and over," said Jayne during her initial consultation with me. "I always gain it back again, plus a few extra pounds. What's wrong with me?"

Like Jayne, many of my patients are veteran dieters. In my work as a psychoanalyst and author specializing in food, weight, and body-image issues, I hear from men and women all over the world who are ready to get off the diet rollercoaster but don't know how. They are fed up with counting calories, carbs, and fat grams, and obsessing over every bite and sip. They lose weight, only to regain it when they start eating normally. Ever hopeful, they try another new diet, only to be disappointed again.

Can you relate? If you're reading this book, it's likely that you have also tried many weight-loss programs. Every year there is a hot new diet craze that promises to melt off pounds by eating this but not that: Paleo, Atkins, South Beach, Cabbage Soup, Cookie Diet, Weight Watchers, and more. They all tell you something different: eat protein, but not carbs. Eat carbs, but not fat. Eat fat, but not carbs. No wonder so many people are confused about health and nutrition—every expert seems to have a different perspective. It's enough to make you want to toss up your hands in defeat.

My friend Fred Cuellar knows exactly how you feel. His personal experience with dieting left him frustrated, baffled, and heavier than before, and he wondered why diets never work in the long run. This led him to seek answers to the question that millions of people ask on a daily basis:

Why can't I lose weight and keep it off?

Fred is a best-selling author and entrepreneur whose success is due in part to his wish to make a difference in people's lives. When he wants to figure something out, he becomes a veritable Sherlock Holmes, immersing himself in research, and he does not stop until he finds the answers. That's why, when Fred decided to solve the mystery of why diets don't work, he started by defining the problem. In the United States alone, it is estimated that 108 million people are on diets at any given time. The diet industry rakes in about $60 billion annually by promising that a thinner, slimmer, happier you is within reach. Each year we spend billions on diet food and diet drinks, yet 37 percent of all Americans are considered obese, and half of Europeans and 63 percent of Australians are considered overweight.

Millions of us are dieting, yet obesity levels keep rising. Why?

Fred was also determined to find a solution to the diet problem. He set out on a mission to create a formula to lose weight permanently, in a way that is easy and sustainable.

And that is exactly what he accomplished in *The Buffer Zone*.

In this groundbreaking book, Fred analyzes the scientific underpinnings of why so many of us struggle with weight. He explains the science behind weight loss and weight gain, while debunking several myths about what we should or should not eat or drink. Using himself as a guinea pig, and with much trial and error, he devised a method to lose weight and maintain a healthy body, all without deprivation, hunger, or willpower. Now, he's sharing the results of his research with you.

You will discover the secret that the diet industry doesn't want you to know: *dieting actually makes you gain weight.* There is a reason that you've been stuck in a discouraging pattern of dieting, losing pounds, and then regaining weight. You haven't failed at dieting. Dieting has actually failed you. The good news is this book will give you the tools to finally enjoy freedom from dieting and achieve your healthiest weight.

The Buffer Zone is not a diet book. You will not be required to measure carbs, count fat grams, or starve yourself. Instead, you will be given a specific method of timing your meals to lose weight and, best of all, keep it off. By putting this technique into practice, you will be attuned to your body in a completely new way and give yourself the nutrition you need to optimize weight loss.

I specialize in the psychology of weight loss, so I appreciate that Fred also recognizes the powerful influence of our minds when it comes to eating problems, and he provides guidelines on how to distinguish physical hunger from emotional hunger. In our culture, we often view our bodies as our primary "selves" and it's important to recognize and value our intellectual, creative, relational, and emotional parts. This book inspires readers to nurture and nourish their minds and souls, as well as their bodies. As Fred puts it, "The goal is not just to lose weight; it's to be healthy."

This is a highly researched, scientifically based, and experientially proven book. Fred Cuellar's personal story adds a compelling vulnerability, and his sense of humor comes through and makes this book fun to read. The discovery of "the buffer zone" is a significant achievement and contribution to the field of weight management, and it will be your last stop on your path to weight loss and good health.

Nina Savelle-Rocklin, PsyD
Author, *Food For Thought: Perspectives on Eating Disorders*
Los Angeles, California

Introduction

I t's already been over a decade since *The New England Journal of Medicine* published the jaw-dropping publication, "A Potential Decline in Life Expectancy in the United States in the 21st Century," and things have gotten worse, not better. The article could easily be summed up in one sentence: if you were born after the year 2000, you are less likely to live longer than your parents. According to figures published in *The Lancet,* since 1980 the worldwide number of obese people has skyrocketed from 875 million to 2.1 billion; in less than thirty years the number of obese people has more than doubled. We are literally eating ourselves into an early grave—an expensive one at that. The estimated healthcare costs associated with obesity in the United States alone are a mind-blowing $190.2 billion a year—practically 21 percent of every dollar spent on medical care.

What are we going to do?

We have to wake up! We have to pull together and realize that we are not powerless against obesity; we just don't understand it. We don't truly understand why our bodies retain fat, lose fat, or gain fat. We don't know the root causes of obesity or how to truly address the issue because we've been told half-truths and whole lies about why we've become a nation that is decaying under its own weight. We have to address the lies and must find the truth. That's what this book is about.

The diet industry rakes in about $60 billion a year! If they can get you to focus on your weight and get you to try their new scheme, your bottom line goes down and theirs goes up. That stops today. Knowing how your body works and being in a stable relationship with food isn't just our goal—it's our mission. The book you are holding has the formula *that regulates weight for the human body*. After reading this book and taking The Buffer Zone journey, you will know—pure and simple—what you need to know so you can be healthy. This book will change your life. You deserve to be healthy. I will show you how.

Here is a brief overview of the contents of this book:

Section I

Chapter 1: F=MA

What we believe has a dramatic effect on how our lives turn out. Our beliefs matter; they chart our course. The sad part is, we've been lied to about why we are fat and furthermore have been told we are to blame for our current state. Chapter 1 examines the top ten lies we've been told about our diet.

Chapter 2: Who Am I? Why Should You Listen to Me?

There's an old riddle: how far can you run into the woods? Answer: halfway, because after that, you are running out of the woods. In chapter 2, I give you the backstory of who I am and where I've been. Before we try to find our way back home, I figured it was important you know a little bit about the man you are trusting to take you through this journey. When you can't see the forest for the trees, you need to know who is going to help you find your way out.

Chapter 3: Stroked Out

Do as I say, not as I did. In chapter 3, I explain the highest price I almost paid for not taking care of my body—my life. Through my bad example of being a person who made everything in his life a higher priority than his health and almost lost it all, I will teach you that it's time to make more time for you.

Chapter 4: Time for Me to Lose

Before I can educate you on the Buffer Zone, I take you back to my first, old-school traditional diet so you can see the classic mistakes we make when we diet. Our mind-set that "suffering" is the only way for a diet to work just isn't true.

Chapter 5: The Revenge of the Body Snatchers

Most people I've met have been on countless diets. Their diets worked initially, quickly stopped working, and then the weight came back with a vengeance! Sound familiar? In chapter 5, I'm forced to slay the dragon of obesity again—but this time the dragon is ready for me.

Chapter 6: Breaking the Code

Chapter 6 explains the three environmental pillars that regulate our mind-body and sets the foundation for the Buffer Zone.

Chapter 7: The Seven Healthy Questions

What are the seven things you need to know in order to be healthy? What are the four laws of weight management? Once we know what to do, we still have to figure out how to do it. If you don't know how your body works, you won't be able to get it to work for you.

Chapter 8: The Equation

This is where all the magic comes together! We define the seven truths of creation and also the unified theory of weight. We may not discover the theory of everything but we find the formula that *regulates weight for the human body*.

Chapters 9 & 10: Guinea Pig, Parts 1 and 2

Once I found the formula that regulates weight for the human body, I had to know its limits. In chapters 9 and 10, I become the guinea pig in my own real-life experiment to see how close I could fly to the sun.

Section II

Chapter 11: Buffer Zone 1 (Your Core)

Let the diet begin! After taking you through my personal voyage of the Buffer Zone in Chapters 1–10, the spotlight is now turned to you, the reader, to implement everything that you've learned and begin getting your life back. Chapter 11 takes you step by step through everything you need to do and is filled with examples of the three core buffer zones you can pick from.

Chapter 12: Buffer Zone 2 (Accelerated Fat Burning)

Ready to take your training wheels off? Chapter 12 shows you how to take your buffer zone to the next level and burn away even more fat! Once you've mastered Buffer Zone 1, Buffer Zone 2 becomes your next challenge.

Chapter 13: Primers and Full Tanks

Food is fuel. What you eat is as important as when you eat. In Chapter 13, I break down all the essential nutrients you need to get through your day.

Chapter 14: Buffer Zone 3 (Maximum Fat Burning)

End of the road? Not hardly. The last few pounds you need to lose are always the toughest. In Chapter 14, we crank up the volume to get you to your weight-loss goal and a new healthy you.

SECTION I

F=MA

n physics, I learned that the force of an object is equal to its mass times acceleration. Mass and acceleration work in inverse proportion to each other; the more mass an object has, the less its ability to accelerate. Conversely, the easier something can accelerate, the less mass it has. Think of light; nothing is faster and look how much mass it had to drop to achieve top speed of 186,200 miles per second.

I promise I'll keep the physics to a minimum, but in this simple and elegant formula, humans are represented by the force and our life is tethered to our mass. Simply put, if our mass gets too big, we won't be able to move. We call this inability to move death. The opposite also holds true: if you are always moving, never slowing down and resting, sometimes your mass will go through mechanical stress in the form of pressure and you will be broken apart through deformation. Your body will collapse due to the strain.

Scary. Move too much and you fall apart, move too little and you fall apart. So, where is the balance?

Maybe another way to look at this formula is as follows:

Fat = My Actions

If I don't pay attention to what my fat is telling me, it could cost me everything.

In search of that balance, let's take a look at all the lies we've been told throughout our lives:

1. Breakfast is the most important meal of the day.
2. The easiest way to lose weight is to eat a lot of small meals.
3. Skinnier people have a high metabolism.
4. Late-night food turns directly into fat.
5. Avoid empty calories; they aren't a source of energy.
6. If you want to lose weight, exercise more and eat healthier.
7. Eat three square meals a day.
8. Fast food is bad food.
9. Avoid fat and carbs.
10. Drink eight glasses of eight ounces of water a day.

Lie #1:
Breakfast is the Most Important Meal of the Day

In a randomized trial published by Cornell University in 2003, researchers in *Psychology and Behavior* found that participants of the study ate approximately 145 more calories at lunch when they ate nothing in the morning versus when they had breakfast. But wait! Considering that the average calorie intake at breakfast is 625 calories, the net savings in calorie intake per day is 480 fewer calories. And 480 fewer calories per day translates into approximately 45 pounds of weight loss in a year!

Now, am I saying that what our mothers told us when we were young—"Always start the day with a healthy breakfast"—is wrong? No. There are no evils here. In fact, there is a significant amount of observational studies that suggest a breakfast high in protein versus a high-sugar/high-carbohydrate breakfast can be beneficial in childhood development for children and teens. But—and here is the big but, if you're an adult reading this and you're trying to maintain a healthy body, breakfast may be the worst thing you can do to start your day! Why? Because eating makes you hungry. The sad part is that it isn't real hunger! Your brain is going to tell you that you've got to get more food because you're "starving" when you really aren't. The folks at Lay's potato chips got it right: "You can't eat just one." Once we take a bite of food our brains crave more. So, knowing when and when not to feed our brains is going to be the key to a healthy you. Knowing your Buffer Zone is going to be the greatest single secret to managing your health than practically anything else you will ever learn. In fact, it may save your life.

Breakfast is a double-edged sword. If you skip it, your body stays in sleep mode (your lowest metabolic rate) and not only does your body burn fewer calories to operate, you're sluggish until it gets fuel. The flip side is once you eat, you've woken up your hunger and will need more fuel in a few hours. Also, it's so easy to overeat at breakfast and eat the wrong foods. Is breakfast the most important meal of the day? No, but you can't skip it or go too big.

Lie #2:
The Easiest Way to Lose Weight Is to Eat a Lot of Small Meals

I can't tell you how long I've heard that eating a lot of small meals—"frequent snacking"—(healthy foods) is a great way to prevent hunger, run a fast metabolism, and control your blood sugar. "Six to eight small meals is the secret to success!" Problem? It's a BIG FAT LIE! I'll repeat it again: EATING MAKES YOU HUNGRY! Why would I want to crank up my appetite over and over again all day long? It's insane!

A study from the University of Ottawa found that on a low-calorie diet there was no weight-loss advantage to divvying up your calories over six or more meals. Another study showed that increasing the number of meals did not boost your metabolism so that you could burn more calories or fat but actually made people want to eat more. Cravings went through the roof! Mozart said it best: "The space between the notes is as important as the notes themselves." In other words, the time you spend not eating between meals is as important as the meals themselves. If those time intervals are too small, you will gain weight. If they are too long, you will get sick. **Determining the proper space**

between your meals is what this book is all about. Finding your Buffer Zone.

Lie #3:
Skinny People Have a High Metabolism

Before we can dispel this old wives' tale, let's be clear what we are talking about when we say metabolism.

Metabolism is derived from the Greek word *metabolē*, meaning "change." It refers to all the chemical reactions in living organisms. Without a metabolism, living organisms (us) would not be able to grow, reproduce, or maintain their form or interact with their environment.

Our metabolism is in charge of breaking down organic matter so we can have the energy to operate our bodies. This is referred to as *catabolism*. Once our bodies use up the available energy that it was given, any extra energy or toxins that our bodies don't burn off get stored as body fat.

The process of building up (muscle and fat) is called *anabolism*. Anabolism is driven by catabolism. Anabolism stores energy, catabolism releases it. Think of a log burning in a fireplace. The log would represent either new food or stored fat from your body. The fire is your metabolism. Its job is to break up the food or fat log and release its energy stores to keep your body running. The key thing to remember—and this is critical—the "fire," your metabolism, never goes out! It's always burning. What it burns is up to you. You can feed it food logs or fat logs. If you only feed it food logs your body will use up the new energy that has been released and store the excess (with its toxins) into stored fat (fat logs).

However, if you balance the scale and burn fat logs sometimes for needed energy, then your fat storage inventory goes down and you get slimmer. People with more lean muscle mass have higher metabolisms (bigger fires) than skinny people with little muscle mass. Bigger people need more energy than little people. So, thinking a person is thinner because they have a faster metabolism is false. If a person is thin, it is just a byproduct of using up all or most of the released energy from food logs and occasionally burning excess fat/toxin logs so they don't gain weight. Sadly, most people are clueless as to how a body actually processes energy and keeps them alive. But that's all going to change. We are no longer going to swallow "beautiful lies" that the food industry feeds us so they can stay wealthy at the cost of our health.

Lie #4:
Late-Night Food Turns Directly into Fat

Regardless of the time of day or night, or how active or sedentary you are, your body is consuming calories. Technically speaking, we all have a basal metabolic rate (BMR), which sets the minimum amount of energy your body requires to stay functioning at rest. There are a lot of systems at work in your body that never get a break. Your liver, brain, heart, and kidneys are just some of the organs that require a 24/7 energy hookup. While the heavy lifting of a digestive system is usually done in three to four hours, a typical digestive system isn't considered inactive until after ten hours. So, when you had your last meal before your late-night snack has more to do with how much fat you pack away than anything else.

For example, let's say the last meal you had before your midnight snack was at noon. Since your quick available energy resources are low, your body is going to gobble up the vittles and turn them into energy to keep your major systems operating. Remember this: *Last In, First Out (LIFO)*. Your body will always grab the newest energy available first to keep the body running.

Here's an analogy that should drive the point home: Everyone has gone shopping for milk at the grocery store; the grocer always restocks the shelves by leaving the oldest in front and placing the newest in the back. This, of course, makes sense because all milk has an expiration date and the grocer wants to sell the older milk first. But that's not how our bodies work. Our bodies take the new food energy and stock our energy shelves from the front instead of the back. Translation: your body will always grab the newest energy first, not the oldest. Fat occurs when our energy requirements are met and there is still too much new energy available. When the supply exceeds the demand, our bodies store fat. It doesn't make a difference what time it is because our bodies are processing plants that are always open. When we sleep, our energy requirements are still 70 percent of what they were during waking hours. Meals or snacks eaten too closely together (too short of a buffer zone) pack the pounds.

Lie #5:
Avoid Empty Calories; They Aren't a Source of Energy

Before we can talk about what an "empty" calorie is or isn't, let's define a calorie. A *calorie* is the approximate amount of energy required to raise the temperature of one gram of water by one degree Celsius at a pressure of one atmosphere. But it's easier to think of a calorie as food energy. When we eat food, our bodies convert food into chemical energy. Food can be broken down into three main groups: carbohydrates, fats, and proteins. Vitamins and minerals can be added to the list but they make up only a small percentage of our food energy.

Now let's look closer: does all food have the same energy density? No. Oh, a new term; let's define it. *Energy density* is the amount of energy stored in a given system or region or space. It's important to remember that while water, minerals, vitamins, cholesterol, and fiber contain virtually no food energy, they are still required for our health and well-being. Fats have the most amount of food energy per mass, followed by proteins and carbs. A portion of fat has over twice as many calories as an equal portion of protein or carbs. That's why fat tastes so good! Our bodies were designed to crave the food that would give us the most energy. Bacon, anyone? So, while it's true that different food groups have different nutritional value, a calorie is still a calorie in its ability to provide energy.

All calories, nutritional or otherwise, have the capability to give us fuel to stay alive. When we hear the word "empty" and attach it to "calorie" it's easy to assume that that calorie has no value, like putting water in your gas tank. Unleaded gas, regular or premium, will run your body. The only difference is some will run it cleaner and leave fewer toxins in you.

Are calories empty? No, not when they are defined as fuel and not nutrition. But here is a good question: does all fuel burn at the same rate? I promise you a fighter jet burns through fuel quicker than your car does, so how much activity (active or inactive lifestyle) can definitely affect how long that calorie gives you energy. Remember the analogy from before about a fire representing our metabolism? Well, the more demand placed on the fire, the more wood it will burn, even if the fire remains at a constant temperature. But what about the calorie logs: are all logs created equal? No. Something called a *glycemic index* lets us know how long a particular type of food will give us energy. Some foods, like potato chips, burn up quickly and immediately dump glucose (sugar) into our bloodstream. Other foods, like starchy vegetables, take a lot longer for our body to break down and supply a steady stream of glucose to your blood versus it being dumped all at once.

Let's go back to the burning firewood analogy. Low glycemic foods are similar to strong dense firewood that can burn for hours. Medium glycemic foods like bananas, orange juice, and ice cream burn up like throwing sawdust on the fire. High glycemic foods like white bread, French fries, and donuts are like pouring gasoline on the fire; big explosion, and then nothing. Calories aren't empty because all calories contain fuel, but if the fuel doesn't last, your body is going to always crave food. So, how long a calorie takes to enter the bloodstream is important. Alcohol by itself is horrible for you, as is a box of donuts. But make a meal cocktail that mixes low- and high-glycemic foods together, we can have our treats (quick-burning fuel) and still have in place some long-burning food logs to keep us from getting hungry thirty minutes after we are done. Win-win.

Lie #6:
If You Want to Lose Weight, Exercise More and Eat Healthier

The purpose of exercise is fitness, not to lose weight. If some minor weight loss is a side effect to being more fit, then great! It's natural to assume when we see an overweight person that they must need to exercise more but the assumption is false. It's possible to be overweight, heck, even obese, and be cardio and muscularly fit. Think of a well-tuned Ferrari pulling a giant U-Haul filled to the brim with heavy bricks. Is the Ferrari fit? Yes. Is its engine in shape? Yes. But clearly dragging around the U-Haul is slowing it down, and eventually it will take a toll on the engine as well as the body. Fat can be fit, but there is more strain on the system. Too much weight comes from too much eating.

And when I say too much eating, it doesn't make a difference if its calories from healthy food or calories from birthday cake. If anyone is overweight, it's because they are supplying more energy than the body is demanding. When the supply exceeds the demand, we gain weight. If we want to be healthy, we don't consume more raw material (food) than our bodies need. If we are Olympic Gold-medalist Michael Phelps, we can gobble ten thousand calories a day because the workload that is being asked of our body is so high. Our food intake must be driven by demand, not the other way around. If we think we can just increase our workload enough to balance the scale, good luck. Last time I checked, an average hour of working out each day burns approximately 557 calories. A single buttermilk biscuit with sausage, egg, and cheese has 670 calories and can be eaten in less than five minutes. Do you really think anyone can use exercise alone without adjusting their food intake and be healthy? Come on, that's nuts! By the way: a small amount of nuts every day is yummy for your body. It supplies wonderful, unsaturated fatty acids and other heart-healthy nutrients—but let's stay on point.

Too little exercise is not healthy; too much exercise is not healthy. As we will discuss later, you will see that finding the perfect balance of exercise will keep you active for your whole life and not just a few days until you hurt yourself. More people injure themselves by over-exercising than by just about any other cause. Another problem with exercising too much is that it makes you HUNGRY! The number of people that end up gaining—not losing—weight by working out more is through the roof because it's just too easy to "overeat" your workout.

Now let's address a healthy diet. When most people try to control their diet through avoidance of "bad" food, they are destined to fail. I have a friend who for years told herself that bread wasn't healthy and must be avoided. She had a chef cook her only healthy food. Did it work? No! She initially lost weight but gained it all back. Why? Because she ate *too much* healthy food! Please get this: when too much food (healthy or not) is placed into the body and not used, it is stored as fat. Ferrari with a U-Haul!

Buffer Zones place more time between meals you love so you can be slim, sexy, and happy. It just turns out that the typical person only needs 7 "full" meals (1,000–1,500 calories each) and 11 "primer" meals (300 calories or less) a week to operate efficiently. The 7/11 Plan. Then consider most people have 14 to 21 "regular" meals (500 or more calories each) and an additional

35 to 49 snacks a week, it's no wonder we are a nation of overweight/obese people. Too many heavy meals equals too many heavy people.

Buffer your meals. Place more time between your eating events and learn to delay gratification and not eliminate it. Instant gratification equals fat. Delayed gratification equals slim, sexy, and healthy. No gratification, or gratification denied, is not only unhappiness but also failure waiting to happen. If you only try to follow a traditional healthy diet and label some foods as bad, you will fail. There are no bad foods, just foods we should eat less of—an important distinction. In our food cocktail, we will show you exactly how to balance comfort food and healthy food so you can have the right octane in your tank! There's light at the end of this tunnel—and it's YOU!

Lie #7:
Eat Three Square Meals a Day

It's always been pretty clear to us that if someone didn't eat for a long enough time, a lot of bad things happened to him/her. Eat or die. What's crazy is we are literally dying now because we eat too much and too often. According to an NBC News report, *Heavyburden: Obesity May be Even Deadlier Than Thought*, obesity and heart disease should be listed as America's number one cause of death. Approximately 598,000 people die each year from heart disease, according to the Centers for Disease Control and Prevention, and obese people are more likely to have heart disease. Two-and-a-half-million people die each year and almost one in four dies because their heart gives out. So what are we supposed to do?

In the Lord's Prayer, we ask God to "Give us this day our daily bread." It doesn't say anything about our breakfast bread, lunch bread, or dinner bread. Daily. Once.

Where did three square meals even come from? If we check the chronicles, we discover that in the 1700s–1800s British and American ships would serve their sailors three full meals on square wooden trays or plates. Being a sailor back then required a ton of calories. Then the European settlers got to America and continued the practice, minus all the sailing, of course. Do you see a weight gain coming? Inactive settlers with three square meals equals chubby settlers. Those habits had been ingrained from being on the ship. When the colonizers first made contact with the American natives they noticed they didn't have a clock to determine when to eat. It appeared the locals only ate when they got hungry and for that we called them savages. They wouldn't conform to society's eating habits. Wow, smart Indians. Eat when you're truly hungry? Genius!

But seriously, think about it. How many times do you look at a clock and go, "Oh, it's *time to eat*!"? I know I used to do it daily. Noon meant it was time for lunch. But we never really ask the bigger question: "Am I actually hungry?" There is such a huge social component around our meals; we feel we don't want to be left out of the fun. So what's the result? We eat when we aren't hungry, we eat when we are hungry, and we eat when we *think* we are hungry.

Did you know that just one hour after any meal your digestive system sends a hormone called ghrelin to your hypothalamus to ask if any more food is coming down the pike? Of course, all the brain understands is, "Hmm, maybe I'm still hungry."

No! If you have had a full meal and your brain is contemplating eating more food, and it's been less than three hours since you last ate, stop! You are getting mixed signals. You aren't hungry; your digestive system is just asking you if you're going to eat more because, if not, it will start its shutdown.

Big cardinal rule #1: Never eat another bite! Not a cookie, not a Hershey kiss, or even a piece of fruit within three hours of your last meal.

This is what I refer to as the Buffer Zone! No eating allowed! The second you start up the digestive system again (and that's easy) you will have fake hunger pains again for up to three hours. EATING MAKES YOU HUNGRY! Remember that. Now, sometimes that can be difficult because the digestive system starts when you merely see or smell food. Crazy, right? There is a solution: just tell yourself, "I ate less than three hours ago. I'm not really hungry." You'll be fine in less than five minutes. Just get away from the stimulus. Because let's be real: if you're sitting in front of a dozen freshly baked, chocolate chip cookies, your digestive system will keep on gurgling. Three square meals a day? Are you a sailor? If not, let's leave it to our daily bread and not three squares.

Lie #8:
Fast Food Is Bad Food

In 2011, John M. Gottman, PhD, wrote the book *The Science of Trust: Emotional Attunement for Couples.* In the book, Dr. Gottman points out predictors of divorce. The one that to this day stands out the most to me is "more negativity than positivity." He found that in healthy, stable relationships the ratio of positive interaction to negative interaction is 5:1. In unhealthy relationships headed for divorce the ratio is 0.8:1. Wow! I thought that data was fascinating. In stable relationships, the couple reported five positive interactions for every one unpleasant one. In the couple headed for divorce court, it was a flip of the coin as to whether the couple would get into a fight every time they interacted with one another. Now, you might be asking, what does this have to do with fast food? Well, everything! I began to wonder if I could apply the same model used in happy relationships to home cooked meals and fast food. Could I eat out at any restaurant once for every five homecooked meals I ate and still maintain my weight or lose weight?

The answer was yes. I shared my idea with others and they had the same results! Is going out to eat where the food is laced with butter, sugar, and salt good for you? Well, yes . . . if it is balanced with homecooked meals. The most important thing I learned was that it is wrong for us to label any food as "bad" and try to avoid it. I found I immediately craved what I couldn't have. When you're hungry and your options are limited, we all know fast food is better than no food. If we monitor the number of times we go for the quick fix, we can stay in this game called Life.

Lie #9:
Avoid Fat and Carbs

The South Beach Diet avoids certain fats and high-glycemic carbs. Atkins tells us to avoid carbs altogether! Both of these fad diets made a lot of money for their creators but, as I pointed out, avoidance is a plan that never works in the long term. We can't help what we like. Some of us have sweet tooths, while others can't pass up a French fry. The secret to successful living is so simple, as you will see when we go over the program in the second half of the book. Excess inventory (fat) is simply a by-product of too much production that exceeds demand. Whether we consume good food, healthy food, or sugary desserts, we are a nation that eats too many meals. We have become calorie counters when we should just be meal counters: we see the trees and not the forest. If we reduce the number of meals we eat, it's amazing how the calories take care of themselves.

Banish the thought that we should avoid anything in our lives, because the second we allow our fears to drive our actions, we might as well check out. At my office, it's always someone's birthday or a holiday (i.e., when society tells us it's okay to have a cheat day). Imagine if we applied that logic to our marriages or our taxes! Would our spouses or the government be so forgiving? We can't continue to eat the same number of meals and snacks and think we can tinker with them or exercise the calories away. It won't work; it hasn't worked.

In studies where animals were limited to eating schedules for only eight to ten hours and then food was restricted for the remainder of the day, those animals lost 35 percent more body fat and lived one-third longer. That sounds good, doesn't it? Avoid anything? Well, yes. Avoid too many meals! If we graze like cows all day eating anytime we want, why should we be surprised that's what we resemble when we look in the mirror?

Lie #10:
Drink Eight 8-Ounce Glasses of Water a Day

In 1945, the Food and Nutrition Board of the National Academy of Sciences published a report in their dietary guidelines that suggested ingesting 2,500 millileters (2.5 liters) of fluid on a daily basis. No clinical study was cited, because no clinical study was ever done. Then, Frederick J. Stare, a nutritionist and founding chairman of the Department of Nutrition at the Harvard School of Public Health, recommended 6 or so 12-ounce glasses of water a day. After a while it got easy to remember "8 and 8", or 8 8-ounce glasses a day. Just because we believe something doesn't make it true. To this day, you can find article after article telling us how many gallons of water we "need" to drink. Even as we sit in our air-conditioned rooms and drink iced tea, the message is clear: Drink More Water! But who is sending out the message?

In an article published in the *British Medical Journal*, Margaret McCartney debunked the eight glasses of water myth and noted that the water advocacy group in Europe Hydration for Health was not only sponsored by but created by food giant Dannon. Dannon sells Volvic, Evian, and Badoit bottled waters, just to name a few. Time and time again we find Big Money behind all the recommendations to eat more food or drink more water. It's so easy to forget that food is a drug. And for two-thirds of us, we are hooked.

It takes 10 percent of our energy to process food and, if we are eating willy-nilly, whenever we want, we will never feel 100 percent full. What if I told you to only put a gallon or two of gas in your car at a time, that it was "healthier for your car" to have six to eight little fill-ups a day. You would think I'm crazy! Eventually you would get that you were wasting too much time worrying about fill-ups to get anything done. You'd break down, do one good fill-up and do your best to increase the time between fill-ups.

The time between fill-ups is a buffer zone. With the right buffer zones between your fill-ups, your car and your body will always have enough energy. The difference with your car is it won't allow you to overfill and your body will. That's why we have to know how to fill up our own tank!

Believe it or not, most people eat until they are stuffed, not until they aren't hungry anymore. How much sense does that make? Eat till it hurts? Insane. How much water should you drink?

The honest experts say there are three easy ways to check:

1. If you're thirsty, drink some water;

2. If you have been exerting a lot of energy and have been sweating a lot, drink some water or even a sports drink to help replace the lost sodium; and

3. Pay attention to the color of your urine. If it is too yellow, drink more water until it turns clear.

It's sad that we can't trust many so-called experts out there who give us health advice. But, sadly, if their opinions have been bought and paid for, they probably aren't worth the price of admission. Over 750 million people don't have access to clear drinking water and Big Food is telling us to overdrink. I've always had two rules for life that have stood the test of time:

1. Take only what you need.
2. Share everything that you've got.

Give love, get love; it's a good formula.

CHAPTER 2

Who Am I? Why Should You Listen to Me?

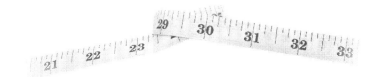

L et's face it: unless you're part of a very small, tight-knit group of people in the jewelry industry, you've probably never heard of me. And that's okay; who I am isn't important. The only thing that is important is that you get to live in a healthy body for as long as is humanly possible. The statement, "If you don't have your health, you don't have anything!" is 100 percent true.

That said, I do believe there is value in understanding how I think and how I've addressed crises and opportunities in the past. I strongly believe it's important to know how and why I came to write this book. That's what this chapter is all about.

The Beginning

I'm told that on April 1, 1963 (I know—April Fool's baby), I was born in the wee hours of the morning to my dad, Lieutenant Hector Cuellar (USAF) and my mom, Elvira Cuellar. I weighed in at eight pounds thirteen ounces. My mom said I looked like a little sumo wrestler. Apparently, I had no trouble getting fed when I was in my mom's tummy. My folks told me that within days of bringing me home I was always screaming for food. Clearly since the umbilical cord was cut I did not have access to a steady stream of nutrients. (That's the thing about babies in the womb; there are no Buffer Zones. Every baby gets what he or she wants, when he or she wants.)

My parents quickly learned that if they wanted peace and quiet, their little baby boy had better be fed every couple of hours. I'm also told that within a week and a half they had to add baby food to the diet because I never appeared satisfied. But for all the troubles of a raging appetite, by all accounts I was still a healthy baby boy.

Life in the Cuellar household went along as I am sure it does in other households. Days turn into weeks, weeks turn into months; a routine is set, and life goes on. We get a little older and hopefully a little wiser. That is, until a few weeks before my third birthday. My mom noticed I had been running a high fever and she put a cool, wet washcloth on my forehead. My mom just assumed I was a little under the weather. When my grandmother came over she touched my little forehead and screamed, "HE'S BURNING UP! We have to get him to the hospital!" Upon arrival at the hospital, my temperature was well over 104 degrees. Doctor

Rodolfo Zaffirini told my folks that if my temperature wasn't lowered, there would be dire consequences. They placed me in a tub of ice water to lower my body temperature. Fortunately, it worked, but they still didn't know what was wrong with me.

Test after test was performed and finally Dr. Zaffirini delivered the bad news: I had spinal meningitis and the prognosis looked bleak. For the first time in my young parents' life they had to face the fact that their happy, bouncing baby boy might not be with them much longer. The plan to help me was straightforward: throw everything at me but the kitchen sink and hope I turned the corner. My heart stopped—not just once, but a few times. Fortunately for me, they were always able to get my ticker going again. My dad recalls a conversation with the doctor where he was told that if my heart stopped one more time, the doctor didn't know if he would be able to get it going again; my dad had to be prepared for the worst. Not long after that, my mom was delivered the news: "Elvira, I'm sorry. Your son has passed away."

I can't imagine how my mom felt at that moment, but I know how I feel when I've been told that someone close to me has died, and there is always a moment of shock and disbelief. The world freezes for a moment. But my mom didn't freeze, she told the doctor to turn around and save her son! As Dr. Zaffirini started to explain that it was too late, that a brain can only go so long without oxygen, she kept screaming, "SAVE MY SON, NOW!" Thankfully, he marched back into my room and paddled my little heart one last time. I came back with a steady sinus rhythm, but I wouldn't wake up.

Dr. Zaffirini now told my parents the likely outcomes. One, I might never wake up from my coma. Two, if I did awaken, I could be blind or brain damaged from the lack of oxygen. Three, if I'm lucky I might be able to keep my sight and only be mentally and physically handicapped. I don't recall if they were ever told that there was much of a chance for a total recovery. I was alive but broken.

My mom stayed by my side, holding my hand and telling me not to give up. She told me later that she knew that the world had big plans for me and it was time to show that I was a fighter. It was two weeks before I finally opened my eyes and said "Spinach." Popeye was my hero, and I knew when Popeye was weak he always ate spinach. My mom said she grabbed and hugged her little Popeye and told me that everything was going to be all right.

My only memories of those events are from the stories my mom and dad told me through the years. By five years old, I was fitted for my first pair of glasses. I was told I would never see well enough to drive a car or fly a plane like my dad. My coordination was horrible. It was so bad that by third grade my dad put me in karate classes so I could learn how to use my body correctly.

In addition, I found that I didn't learn like everyone else. When I was in class, I always had more questions. I annoyed the teachers so much that they would eventually ask me to lower my hand because I was slowing the class down. My sixth-grade math teacher, Mr. Tonack, realized I had a rabid curiosity and fed me brain teasers and allowed me to get extra credit for them. I remember one time he gave me a puzzle (unbeknown to me, it had no solution) to see how I would handle the impossible. And while I can't remember for the life of me what the puzzle was, I do remember working on it day and night. When I finally turned in my answer, Mr. Tonack studied my "answer," only to say he couldn't argue with my conclusion. He gave me an 'A' because he couldn't prove me wrong or right.

I've always loved puzzles. I've always loved knowing how something works. To me, problems weren't problems, they were opportunities to learn the unknown. And since the unknown has always scared me, I've always searched for more answers.

Blackjack

In the summer of 1977, my dad was transferred to Montgomery, Alabama, to attend the Air War College. We lived in a small town outside of Montgomery called Prattville. As a freshman in high school, I was still trying to figure out in what direction I should take my life.

One day, a segment on *60 Minutes* came on TV called "Beat the Dealer." It was all about a man called Dr. Edward Thorp who had written a best-selling book on how to beat the game of blackjack. His proposition was straightforward enough; before a card is dealt, the probability of knowing what cards will come up are all random. But—and this is an important but—if one paid attention to the cards as they are dealt and discarded and kept a running count to what had been played, the player's knowledge of what was left in the deck goes up. And when one's knowledge goes up, the player could adjust their bet accordingly. In blackjack speak, it's called a plus-minus count.

To put it as simply as possible, when a lot of little cards have been played, the deck is rich with high-value face cards. When a lot of face cards have been played, the deck's value goes down because the deck only has a bunch of little cards left that make bad combinations. What Dr. Thorp said fascinated me. It was possible to improve your odds in the future if you paid attention to your previous and present experiences. At the time, I got so excited about being a professional blackjack player that I bought Dr. Thorp's book and Epstein's book on statistical logic and ended up spending the next few years, over five-thousand hours, practicing blackjack. I loved the idea that I could have some control over my future. While I didn't realize it at the time, there are a lot of similarities between knowing how to sit out of a hand of cards and knowing when not to eat. More on that later.

College

When I got to college, I continued practicing blackjack in my spare time but I was still like any other red-blooded male: I wanted a girlfriend. At Texas A&M, it was a big deal to have a date at Aggie football games. Mostly, because of a wonderful tradition that when the Aggies scored, so did you; you got to kiss your date! Only problem? The freshman women only wanted to date upperclassmen. It seemed no matter how hard I had tried, I couldn't get a date to the coveted Aggie football game. I would set up shop at breakfast at a cafeteria, fill my tray with a bowl of Captain Crunch, and spot any attractive young lady sitting alone.

It didn't work. I kept striking out; even the girls who didn't have a date yet said no because they were holding out for a bigger, better deal. Another perk to being an upperclassman was that they got better seats at the game. Finally, I decided to ask around: did I have a personal problem or was my problem universal to other incoming freshmen? As it turns out, it was a universal problem, and not only among the male freshmen but also among the female freshmen. This didn't make any sense. Here were two groups of people with the same goal and neither one was finding success.

Then it hit me. Ah-ha! This is a problem! And I love problems because hidden in every problem is an opportunity. How could I get these groups coupled off and find a hidden pearl for me? I reviewed some beliefs:

1. To the degree you help others you will be helped, the *Law of Reciprocation.*

2. We tend not to want what we have and desire what we can't have, *the Want Dichotomy.*

I then realized, if women and men got to meet people they believed were perfect matches for them, they would be more likely to take a chance on a date. Even then I knew that all of us are more likely to avoid the unknown (regardless of how much reward comes with it) for the fear of being hurt. As a species, we will always do more to avoid pain than to receive pleasure. If I could remove the pain from finding Mr. or Miss Wonderful, I could get everyone together and we could all be one big happy family. If I knew what people desired, their likes and dislikes, I could easily play matchmaker.

So, what did I do? I went to the computer lab (those were the days when one computer took up a whole room) and asked the teacher if he could run stat sheets for me to find patterns.

"Patterns?" he asked. "Computers are great at finding patterns, but it will be your job to figure out what the patterns mean."

I said "No problem!" then I went from dorm room to dorm room and gave the following pitch:

"Hi, I'm Fred Cuellar, and I've started the very first computer dating company here at Texas A&M. It's called 'Relation Makers.'" I then gave them my card. "If you take just a few minutes to fill out what your likes and dislikes are and what you value in a mate, I will run the data through the school's computer and I will give you the top five matches and their phone numbers. For the price of my service all I charge is a single dollar. What do you have to lose? Isn't a dollar worth possibly meeting the love of your life?"

Did they go for it? Yep! In droves! It didn't take very long before everyone signed up. And not just once—if the first matches didn't work out, they would keep playing the lottery over and over. Everything was coming up roses. I had more money than I ever had in my life, I made enough contacts to have a steady girl, and everyone called me the Dating Guy. I came to A&M a scared, lonely kid hoping someone would like me and now I felt like a player. But the thing about fortune is that sometimes just as quickly as it comes, it evaporates. When the school figured out I was running a business on campus, they shut me down. From rags to riches and back to rags. But I was still counting my blessings; at least I still had a girlfriend, and wasn't that the goal from the beginning?

By age thirty-five, after running a successful business, I was sleeping approximately four hours a night; I worked from sun up until past sundown. My logic was that if a few hours of work made me some greenbacks, more hours of work would make me more money! I was violating the Less is More law. I was spending less time with my friends and family and beautiful wife, LaTeace. Indeed, I had devoted all my time to my work. I was eating on the run. I consumed pure octane (high-fat) meals. My weight was ballooning. And while the extra work did initially bring in more dollars, I couldn't see what burning the candle at both ends was doing to me. The thing about a candle that is lit on both ends is it may burn twice as bright but for only half as long. I was on a dead-end road and never saw the freight train that was about to bring my life to a screeching halt!

CHAPTER 3

Stroked Out

"Open your eyes," I heard a woman say. "Please, honey, for me. Open your eyes."

I opened my eyes. I looked around the room. I was in what appeared to be a hospital room. There was this beautiful woman who looked very concerned standing over me holding my hand. *Wow!* I thought, *She must be a nurse, but she's not dressed like one.*

The sun was coming in through the window; it cast a beautiful amber light across my bed. "Oh my God!" the beautiful woman said. "You're back! You're back!" She started crying and hugging me. "You had us all so worried. Your parents just went down to the cafeteria for a cup of coffee but they will be back in just a few minutes. Oh my God, I love you so much! Don't ever scare me like that again!"

I attempted to say the first thing that came to my head but no words came out. I started getting scared and my eyes started watering. I tried to speak again. Again, nothing. Panic set in. Who is this woman? Why am I in the hospital? How did I get here? What's going on!? I want my mom!

When it became apparent that I couldn't speak, the most beautiful woman in the world said, "Oh my God, you can't speak. Okay, okay, wait. Let me find something to write with." She dug through her purse and found a pen and scratch sheet of paper, which looked like a grocery list on the other side. "Here, write on here. Can we communicate this way?"

I grabbed the piece of paper and laid it out on a side pull-out tray attached to the bed. I wrote, "Who are you?" A look of shock came over the mystery woman and tears ran down her face. I didn't like seeing her cry. I wrote again, "I don't mean to make you cry. If you could just tell me who you are and how I got here that would be great." She pushed the tray out of the way and tearfully said, "I'm your wife! I'm your wife, LaTeace! Don't you remember me? We've been married for ten years! You have to know that!"

The first thought that popped into my head was "Cool! Oh my God! I don't know what world I'm living in or if this is even a dream, but if it is, I don't want to wake up. I'm married to the most beautiful woman in the universe!" At that moment, my folks walked into the room holding coffee and what looked like a danish. I love danish! But, wait, what happened to my parents? They are old. How did my parents get old? What's going on? I want to wake up from my dream now. I have to wake up.

I closed my eyes really hard and wiped the tears away with my arm. I slowly opened my eyes again and looked up; my parents were still old. The beautiful woman claiming to be my wife was still there. I started crying again.

"It's okay, son, it's going to be all right. The doctors think you may have had a stroke. When you passed out you hit your head pretty hard but you're safe now. Everything is going to be okay."

I heard the sound of a phone ringing and it appeared to be coming from my dad's pocket. He reached into his pocket and pulled out a small, clam-like device, like something from Star Trek. A communicator. "Elisa, your brother is fine," my dad said. "It appears he's had a stroke but he's awake now. We are in Room 217 at Saint Luke's Hospital. I'm sure your brother would love to see you."

He closed the communicator. I reached over the table for the paper and pen so I could write. LaTeace moved it closer to me. I wrote, "What is that thing you're talking into?" My dad laughed, "It's a cell phone, silly!" I didn't know what a cell phone was. Then I saw a chart next to my bed that apparently gave instructions to the day nurses and noticed the date. What?! I quickly scribbled on the paper, "What year is it?"

My dad replied, "Well, 1998, of course." I sank in my bed. My last vivid memory was May 25, 1977. I was fourteen years old. What has happened to the last twenty years of my life?

Actions Speak Louder than Words

Back when I was at Texas A&M, like I'm sure a lot of freshmen students, I was required to take Psychology 101. It seemed fair enough to me. The psych professor said on the first day that we were going to take a voyage into the human mind. I joked, "I don't mind," and the professor promptly told me to "keep quiet!" I guess we could learn about the human mind but we couldn't speak our minds. Anyway, there was one particular class that did pique my interest: it was the day we talked about *cognitive dissonance*. Wikipedia defines it like this:

COGNITIVE DISSONANCE

Cognitive dissonance is the mental stress or discomfort experienced by an individual who holds two or more contradictory beliefs, ideas, or values at the same time, performs an action that is contradictory to one or more beliefs, ideas, or values, or is confronted by new information that conflicts with existing beliefs, ideas, or values.

It is believed that humans crave internal order; and when humans experience anything that contradicts their internal order they feel compelled to remove it from their lives.

Let's use an example of you at home in an air-conditioned house. You believe that the temperature inside your home should be set at seventy-one degrees. That makes you feel good. But then your spouse comes along and complains it's too cold in the house. This of course frustrates you because you are all nice and comfy and you might even say to your spouse, "Hey, if you're cold, put on more clothing. As you can see, I'm already in my skivvies and it's not like I have much more to take off!"

Then your spouse sulks, complains, and then throws an extra blanket onto the bed. Okay, stay with me, you got to keep the temperature of the house the way you like it but now your spouse is mad at you. And since one of your beliefs is to keep your significant other happy, you are at an impasse. The house temperature belief is conflicting with the "happy wife, happy life" belief. This is cognitive dissonance. What to do? Well you have a couple choices:

1. Change your belief about keeping your loved one happy (fat chance), or

2. Adjust what temperature you are willing to live with.

The answer seems obvious: if we want to remove the dissonance, change your ideal temperature belief. So, you say to your spouse, "Okay, all right, fine! I'll raise the temperature one degree! But that's it!"

"That would be great," she says, and she moves closer to you. Peace and harmony have been restored. Except now that you're cuddling you're even hotter than you were before—but hey, it's not a perfect world. It beats the cold shoulder.

My point is, mentally and physically we exist in an environment and there is disorder. If our actions don't coincide with our belief systems, there will be chaos. And if there is chaos long enough, you may just wake up in a hospital having survived a stroke and wondering where the last twenty years of your life went, because that's exactly what happened to me.

Your Reflection Doesn't Lie

Panicked and afraid, I tried to talk again but nothing came out. I grabbed the piece of paper and, using all available space left, I wrote, "I want to see a mirror!" There was a mirror by the sink but I had so many monitors and lines running into me, it was clear I couldn't get up.

LaTeace reached into her purse for a small compact, opened it, and handed it to me. As I gazed into that two-by-two-inch little square mirror I saw a grown-up man with a full beard that I had never seen before. If I was awake, and I believed I was, I did not know this reflection in the mirror, even though I knew it had to be me. I remember feeling extremely faint as all the energy left my body. The last thing I remembered was hearing the compact mirror shatter after it fell out of my hand.

* * *

When I opened my eyes again, I noticed that the room was dark except for a light over the head of my bed. The sun was no longer coming through the window and the room was empty except for my wife. Wow. It was still amazing to me that I had grown up and gotten married. I must have done something right in my life to have attracted such a beautiful soul to love me. Regardless of anything else, I couldn't be that big of a loser.

On the shelf by the window was a row of flowers. Vase after vase of beautiful flowers. "Get well soon!" "Hang in there!" "Our hopes and prayers are with you!" the cards read. I didn't recognize the names on the cards. Other people loved me. I kept repeating the people's names on the cards over and over to myself in my head; I wanted so badly to get my memory back.

"Honey, you're awake! Your mom and dad needed some rest, so they went home. Don't worry about anything. I'm not going anywhere.

"The doctor said while it's unusual to have memory loss due to the stroke or hitting your head, he said not to worry. He also said I can show you pictures of our life, like from our wedding and vacations and birthdays and Christmases. They might trigger your memory back. He said we just have to be patient."

I nodded.

"Also, I've got a fresh pad of paper and pens so we can talk as much as you like."

I wrote, "Thank you."

"You're welcome," she said and started tearing up. "Oh my God, I promised myself I wouldn't cry!" She grabbed a tissue from the side table and dabbed her eyes. "We are going to get through this. You and me! We're a team; we have always been a team and we can deal with anything! Don't you worry! Do you feel like seeing some pictures of the adventure we've had up until now?" I wrote to say that I did.

I couldn't remember taking any of those pictures.

I wrote, "I'm scared; what if I lose more memory?"

LaTeace looked shocked as she read my words; apparently, it hadn't dawned on her that not only might I not get better but I might get worse. I knew all too well that when growth stops, decay begins.

The Pleasure Principle

Epicureanism is a philosophy on the teachings of ancient Greek philosopher Epicurus. It dates back to 307 BC. A while ago. Epicurus believed that "pleasure" was the greatest good and the key to pleasure was to limit one's desires. He believed that only if you consumed and lived modestly could you ever attain tranquility. He further taught that if you could limit the number of your desires, that not only would the desires that came to fruition have more meaning but you would also be released from the fear associated with consumption. If we believe that our happiness is dependent on acquiring "more," then we are unhappy with our present circumstances. If we are unhappy with our present circumstances, we will tend to fear or lend blame to the things, experiences, and people in our lives. Fear becomes our God and we believe acquisitions are our salvation. (*Note:* If you aren't happy before you acquire anything, you won't be happy after you acquire the thing you "desire.") More leads to less happiness.

Epicurus believed in setting limits on desires because he saw far too well what happened to those who set no boundaries on the desires they had. The dichotomy of desire is so simple; attempting to quench many desires leaves you with less energy/happiness than focusing on a select few that have deep meaning to you. You might have five-thousand Facebook friends, but I bet you figured out long ago that you can probably count your true friends on one hand.

While many have interpreted Epicurus's work as an attempt to avoid pain, nothing could be further from the truth. The avoidance of all pain and seeking only pleasure is hedonism, and it doesn't ever lead to a happy ending (although it does lead to your ending). Epicurus was ahead of his time; he understood full well that it took a lot of hard work and yes, pain, to limit one's desires so they could mean more to you and so that you could have a meaningful life.

So many people nowadays see the pleasure principle as twofold: seek pleasure, avoid pain. The irony in this herculean task is the attempt to avoid all pain is the greatest pain of all. In avoidance, we find pure unadulterated pain. In our attempt to remove everything, everyone, or every experience that is painful, we are led down a dark path where we find the only one left standing in the room is ourselves. That's how we came into this world and how we go out. The time in between is to make connections, to honor desires, make commitments, set goals, and have values that define our character.

What is the pleasure principle? If it is defined like Epicurus meant it to be defined, it would be to choose fewer things we want so they mean more to us. Fewer acquaintances for a few real friends. Fewer promises for a few solid commitments. Less talking for a few good actions. Epicurus understood that we are not only defined by the actions that we take but the actions we stop ourselves from undertaking. Again, Epicurus was ahead of his time.

Breaking the Silence

"Where's my husband?" LaTeace asked the day nurse.

"They've taken him for an MRI; he should be back within the hour," she replied.

Teace waited patiently for my return when she heard a very familiar voice coming from down the hall.

"Hi, Wife!" I exclaimed as I was coming in the door being pushed in a wheelchair by an orderly.

"Mrs. Cuellar, looks like your husband is getting better. He just started talking when he was in the middle of the brain scan. It actually took us a while to shut him up and be still," explained the orderly.

"Hi, Honey!" I said. "Can I call you, 'honey'? It just seems right being that we are all married and stuff."

"Of course you can," Teace replied. "So do you remember me? Is your memory back?"

"No," I said, "but it sure feels good to talk again. Not having a voice sucks. Where are my folks?" I asked.

"They just called and they'll be here in an hour. They'll be so excited to know you're talking.

"Sooo . . . there must be something new you remember," Teace said.

"No, not really. I kinda feel like a kid trapped in a grown-up's body," I said.

"You mean like the movie *Big* with Tom Hanks?" she asked.

"Never heard of it," I said.

"What was the last movie you remember?" she asked.

"*Star Wars*! Coolest movie ever! I mean, besides *The Godfather* or *Godfather II*. Classics!" I exclaimed.

"You know—well, I guess you don't—they made *Godfather III*," she said.

For the next few hours, I was caught up about the world. Movies, presidents, cell phones, the Internet. It all sounded like such a brave new world. My mom and dad showed up and I couldn't get over how they had aged. I kept asking about my mom's hair, asking her how it got traded for this gray? In fact, it bothered her enough that she went out and got her hair dyed to look a little younger for me. Before long, I talked myself out and fell asleep.

The body is the most mysterious and wonderful thing in the world. I remember once being asked a riddle, that if I was at home in the middle of the night and the house caught on fire, what would be the one possession I would grab if I only had time to grab one? Most people say they would grab photographs or important papers like passports. There is only one correct answer if you want to live: you take your body out of there! You see, your body is your most prized possession. There is no place we can go to get another one if we lose the one we have.

With my stroke, I was quickly realizing how tough life would be if I didn't have a functioning body. It was bad enough that the right hemisphere stroke had damaged the left side of my body, but I sure didn't ever want to do anything again that would put my body at risk. Fortunately for me, I had time. Time, as it turns out, is the key to everything. While I didn't know it, every second I was in Saint Luke's Hospital my body was fast at work trying to heal itself. Bodies don't like to be broken. Time brought my voice back. Time would bring the use of my limbs back and, yes, time would bring my memories back. Time would heal my wounds.

Survival Instinct

There's an old joke about two campers who are sitting around a campfire in the woods. As the story goes, a bear suddenly appears out of nowhere and rushes the two unsuspecting campers. Startled and horrified, they both get up and start running! As they run for their lives, one of the campers realizes one of his shoe laces had become untied. Knowing that this was slowing him down, he comes to an abrupt stop and kneels to tie his shoe. The other camper, horrified at the prospect of becoming a Big Mac meal for the fast-approaching bear, screams, "Get up! Get up! We have to outrun the bear!" The kneeling camper, after he had finished tying up his laces, remarks, "I don't have to outrun the bear. I just have to outrun you!" He takes off, leaving the other camper frozen in his tracks.

That, in a very simplified way, is what a survival instinct is all about. When we sense we are in danger, our brains are designed to get us to quickly come up with a plan to restore our safety. Fear doesn't just make us feel uncomfortable, it makes us feel unsafe. And once someone feels that their safe place is gone, they will do anything to get it back. Our initial response to an unknown stimulus is to freeze and hyper focus our attention on the assailant or situation that is making us feel uncomfortable. Sometimes freezing works; while we are stuck in "deer in the headlights" mode we are given an opportunity to take in more data to see if we are seriously threatened. When confronted with a loss of safety, our second defense mechanism is to run—also known as the flight response.

That's what the campers did. They didn't stick around and ask the bear what his intentions were, they just headed for the hills. Probably a smart move. There is a quote I heard growing up that I think is appropriate here: "We only run away from the things we fear." It makes sense; why run away from anything we love? That would be silly. But what is interesting is what we learn when we study fear. When we stop to ask where fear comes from, the picture becomes quite clear. We fear what we do not understand. Well, that kind of makes sense and kind of doesn't. If we fear anything we don't understand and then run from it, how can we conquer our fears? And wouldn't this leave us running for the rest of our lives? Every time we turn around we are confronted with things we don't understand.

Now, I'm not saying that we need to give a nice, big ol' bear hug to the rushing bear, but I am saying that most things we don't understand aren't man-eating bears. They're misunderstood conversations with loved ones, or new projects our boss drops on our desk when we thought our workload was already fulfilled to capacity. No, the "bears" in our lives tend to simply come to us through the natural evolution of change. The old biblical quote, "This too shall pass," says it all; they are the words that the happy man doesn't want to hear and yet the sad man does.

While our survival instinct, or better said, our programming for self-preservation, got us where we are today, it doesn't seem to have done much for climate change or the random senseless school shootings that seem to be commonplace in the news these days. It turns out that having a survival instinct is great if you're living in the woods and battling the environment, but lousy when we have to navigate the regular comings and goings in our lives.

One final way of coping is with the other half of "flight or fight" response: to fight. When we finally feel desperate enough, when stopping to ask questions doesn't provide the answers we require for safety, when we've run everywhere we can run but can't find anywhere to hide, we will fight for our survival. The problem is that most of us don't know how to fight. And if you've never learned how to deal with the opponent you're confronted with, your last and final chance for safety will be lost. It is without a doubt that we have an instinct to survive, but believing a box of donuts downed with a soda pop will bring back the comfort we require is wrong. The donut isn't safety; it's the bear.

Just in Time

In 1972 singer-songwriter Jim Croce released the song "Time in a Bottle." In the song, he talks about never having enough time to do the things we want to do and that when we get lucky enough to find the one we want to spend time with, there's never enough time to spend with him or her. If we could only put time in a bottle so that we could save all those precious moments for the ones we love. Such a brilliant song.

Jim Croce lost his life on September 20, 1973, when his chartered airplane crashed and killed him along with five others. Jim Croce was only thirty years old. Nobody knows how much time they get to play with once they arrive on the planet. Croce was right; there never seems to be enough time to do the things you want to do once you find them. That's what makes how we spend our time so special.

I was spending all my time working and no time taking care of my body; my body of work grew while my actual body suffered. We, as a people, aren't very fond of our bodies, and its mostly because no one really taught us how to truly take care of them. We never got a body handbook. Well, that is until now. Once I walked out of that hospital on my own two feet (they like to wheel you out for insurance reasons), I promised myself, even if it takes the rest of my life, I was going to figure out how to take care of the most precious thing I would ever own—my body.

I have spent the last seventeen years since my stroke working on this puzzle called the human body. My journey has taken me through a lot of winding turns and a lot of dead ends, but at just about the time I wanted to give up, I discovered the secret that not only saved my life but could potentially save the lives of millions. It's time to tell you how I turned my life around.

CHAPTER 4

Time for Me to Lose

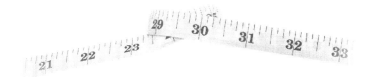

Hurdle #1

There are countless ways to describe an overweight person: big-boned, weight-challenged, thick, husky, large, extra-large, obese, and, of course, simply fat. After my near-death experience with my stroke, I was now facing a brand-new challenge. I was 50 pounds overweight. I tipped the scale at over 235 pounds. Interesting fact: How many 250-pound men over the age of 80 do you think there are on this planet? Answer: zero. If you are a 250-pound, 80-year-old male, please come forward. I'd like to let the experts know you exist.

Anyway, at 235 and coming off a stroke, it was clear that I had to make a lifestyle change. That's what they call it when some expert tells you that you are doing everything wrong in your life: You must make some lifestyle changes. I suppose that sounds better than, "Listen, you either stop stuffing your face and exercise more or the next stroke you have will kill you."

I think I respond better to soft love than to tough love. My weight issue seemed pretty straightforward: change my diet, eat less "bad food," and work out more, and the weight will fall off like leaves from a tree in autumn with a cool breeze.

The first thing I did was get a subscription to *Men's Health* magazine. I felt I might as well follow a proven path than attempt to stumble around in the dark. I immediately loved reading my new fitness bible. It was chock full of wonderful articles designed to help me take care of me: "Eat This and Not That," "How to Have a Six-Pack," "How to Drop that Belly Fat," and "How to Power Up Your Life."

Their first big tip told me that I needed to get rid of all temptations. So, I grabbed a large garbage bag and filled it with all my comfort food: Cheetos, Pop Tarts, Oreos, potato chips, SpaghettiOs, and countless other prepacked, overly processed "evil" foods.

I asked a good friend of mine if he wanted my Santa Claus-filled sack of snacks and he immediately responded, "Sure! Why ya throwing out all your goodies?"

I said, "Oh, haven't you heard? These are 'evil foods,' and if I keep eating them I will get more obese and have another stroke and die! So, I thought you might like to have them."

He said, "You want to give me all the food that is slowly killing you so that you can live a longer and healthier life?"

"Exactly!" I exclaimed.

"Sounds good to me," my buddy replied. "I'm not worried about being healthy! No sense good food going to waste. That would just be criminal."

"That's what I thought, too!" I agreed.

Once I cleared my living environment from temptations, I needed to restock my pantry with all the healthy food listed in my Health Bible. They were mostly low-glycemic foods like starchy vegetables, peanuts, yogurt, and fruits. I was shocked at how easy this was going to be. Eat right + exercise more = healthy me. I imagined that all those weight-challenged people must just have low willpower. But not me!

I copied a workout from *Men's Health* that I could follow every day and, according to my goals, I should be able to lose two to three pounds a week. By my calculations I should hit my goal weight in five months. That's not so bad. Thirty-five years on the wrong path and just five months to self-correct! "Wow," I thought to myself, "being fat is a choice. I'll have this licked in no time!" Boy, I was in for a rude awakening.

Day 1

My *Men's Health* Nutrition System was as follows (this plan can currently be found in the Men's Health Diet: 27 Days to Sculpted Abs and Maximum Muscle):

Fiber-rich grains	**L**egumes
Avocados, oils, & healthy fats	**E**ggs & Dairy
Spinach & leafy greens	**A**pples and fruits
Turkey & Lean Meats	**N**uts & Seeds

F.A.S.T & L.E.A.N. (clever)

+ High-quality protein, mood-boosting folate, brain-building omega-3s, and fiber-rich carbs like whole fruits & vegetables.

– Refined carbs, salt, high-fructose corn syrup & other sweeteners, and trans fats.

The *Men's Health* system told me to stop counting calories. What a relief! Instead, I was to pay attention to loading my plate correctly with nutrient-dense food. Made sense. This is how they told me to pack my plate.

Meats: Size of my palm *(Damn! I thought, Why couldn't I have bigger hands?!)*

Vegetables & Fruits: As big as a closed fist

Oils & Other Healthy Fats: A teaspoon. And a teaspoon was equal to the end of my thumb, from the knuckle up.

Legumes: I had no idea what these were, but apparently I could have a palm's worth.

Grains: Size of a closed fist

Dairy: The size of my palm

I was allowed to have five meals a day. Hmm, this was going to be tricky. I was more of a skip breakfast, fast lunch, heavy dinner, and nighttime snack kind of guy. I was also allowed beverages/desserts but they had calorie restrictions. In fact, every meal had a calorie restriction. They were as follows:

Breakfast: 500–750 calories

Snack: 200–300 calories

Lunch: 400–500 calories

Snack: 200–300 calories

Dinner: 500–600 calories

+ Beverages & Dessert: 200 calories

Ugh, this was going to be tough. But as my father said a million times when I was growing up, "Nothing ventured, nothing gained." Although, I hoped in this case that with this diet venture, I wouldn't gain anything: I would lose, lose, lose weight!

After going to the grocery store, I started preparing myself for my new routine. I bought everything on the recommended food list and by the afternoon of Day One, I was loaded for bear.

You see, my Day One was really more of a preparation day. My "official" Day One was actually the next day. Since I knew I was going to be on a calorie-restricted diet for some time, I felt I would have my final Last Supper. Or, maybe more of a final meal of a death-row inmate. But, either way, I wanted a "splurge day" before I began my sentence. And the way I was going out was with my Boo's (nickname for my wife) homemade lasagna. Yummy, yummy! My mouth salivates thinking about it now.

Yep, I was going to eat all the lasagna I could and top it off with old-fashioned chocolate sheet cake. My last supper was on my terms. All my future suppers would no longer be in my control. While I wasn't aware of it, I was one day away from allowing food to control my life, my every waking thought.

Day 2 (a.k.a., the Real Day 1)

When I was a kid, I would get a nervous energy on the days leading up to the first day of school. I would count down my last days of freedom by staying up late past my bedtime and eating midnight snacks composed of bowl after bowl of Captain Crunch cereal. Occasionally, I'd make strawberry shakes as long as everyone else was awake, as the blender was quite loud. There would be our annual trip for school supplies when I'd figure out what binders, pencils, and loose-leaf paper I'd need for my upcoming journey. I'd buy a protractor, regardless of how much I'd actually use it, because you never knew when you might be asked to draw a perfect circle.

The night before the first day of school I hardly slept. I couldn't; I was too anxious. I kept worrying whether I would get to school on time, where all my classes were, if I would get lost, and what I would be required to do in gym class. I was a late bloomer so I wasn't fond of gym class or any other place that made me undress in front of others. I didn't have any body hair until I was a junior in high school. I found the whole thing quite embarrassing. So, I didn't really sleep; I just kind of lay in bed staring at the alarm clock until it was time to wake up. Even the alarm clock scared me; it was so loud it could wake the dead. I was convinced that one day I would be the youngest person to die from a heart attack because I was startled to death by the clanking, ear-piercing alarm, so I made a point of turning it off before it had a chance to scare me.

The first day of my diet I revisited all those new school year jitters. I didn't sleep; I was so anxious to get started. It's funny, while I knew how many calories I was allowed to have at each meal, I really had no idea how small 500 calories was. For example: A plain bagel with cream cheese is approximately 525 calories. A large Belgian waffle with 1½ tablespoons of maple syrup is 500 calories. A McDonald's Big Mac, four slices of bacon, a Starbucks venti caramel Frappuccino are 500 calories *each*. My God, even a 6-inch black forest ham on wheat bread with oil & vinegar (no cheese toppings) from Subway is 500 calories! What had I signed myself up for? How was I going to survive in a world where the average number of calories for a meal is 1,500? Was I going to live on one-third of that for each meal? It was insane!

Okay, Okay. It's only day one. Take it one meal at a time. You're smart, I told myself. *You're tough. You can do it.* I felt better. This little voice inside of me was kind and encouraging. It was just what I needed.

I opened the refrigerator for a breakfast I normally skipped and pulled out a hard-boiled egg, a small bowl of fruit, and prepared some oatmeal. That's when another, meaner voice in my head chimed in, "This is crazy! Why should I eat when I'm not hungry? Aren't I trying to lose weight? This doesn't make sense!" I missed the kind voice that just moments before told me that I could do this. I tried to just ignore the voices in my head and eat my breakfast. I couldn't believe I hadn't even made it through Day One and was already arguing with myself, an argument that was far from its tipping point.

The Hero's Journey

As someone who had rarely eaten breakfast, a funny thing happened when I did. I awoke a sleeping giant! It turns out, within an hour or two of eating breakfast, I was hungry again! Where did this come from? I used to go all morning and into early afternoon without even giving food a second thought and now here I was, seemingly minutes after eating a breakfast I didn't even want, hungry for more food! Damn! Wait, I had a midmorning snack! The diet gods must have anticipated that my bloodstream would love free-floating glucose (from Greek, meaning sweet wine) or sugar in my veins. It's crazy; I almost felt like I was allowing myself to get hooked on something and now I needed another fix! Regardless, that's why I had a sliced-up Fuji apple. I gobbled it up. Only two more hours until lunchtime.

When twelve thirty rolled around, I pulled out my precooked, lean chicken breast, some nuts, and more Fuji apple. I inhaled it. I would get another snack before three and then a perfectly measured dinner at five thirty.

Food was all I could think about. There was the pizza my coworkers asked if I wanted in on; there were the smells of seafood gumbo coming from the lunchroom (a leftover from a previous night's dinner that my assistant had warmed up) all smelled delicious . . . but I had to say no. I was in a food-deprived hell. When I got home I scarfed my wafer-thin meal like a Triscuit with a dab of Cheez Whiz that was demolished in one bite.

This was horrible. I never felt full. I never felt satisfied. I wasn't having meals, I was having evil temptations that left me feeling hollow, empty, and hungry. Maybe now I understood what it meant to be fat and happy.

But is fat really happy? I wondered. You might be for a split second when you consume the food, but I knew the satisfaction was short-lived. It was quickly replaced by guilt of being a loser for not sticking with my goals, for being a wimp with no willpower. No. No. Fat wasn't happy but neither was Fat on a Diet. All I could think about was the day I would lose these fifty pounds so I could return to my normal life. It might take months but once I got my slim and sexy self back, I would never allow myself to get in such a bind again. I would set weight limits so the second I went over my max weight I'd just shift into diet mode for a few days and then—bada bing!—back on track! Yeah, this first part of the journey would be tough but I had to stick to my guns. Tomorrow was my first official weigh-in and I knew I must have lost one thousand pounds.

Okay, maybe I'm exaggerating a little, but my payoff was going to be my scale. I could already imagine it now. "Hi, Fred—I mean, is that even you?" my scale would say. And no I don't have a talking scale, but this was my fantasy so allow me a little creative license. I would answer my scale and say, "Hi, Mr. Scale! I know I must be difficult to recognize but, yes, it's me. I know why there is some confusion; you see, I've been on a diet for the last twenty-four hours and that's why you're having a hard time recognizing me."

"That's it exactly!" my scale would exclaim. "You mean you've only been on the diet for a day?! Impossible! You look so good!

In fact, why don't you just step up so I can tell you the good news. You like good news, don't you?"

I would enthusiastically reply, "I do, I do!"

"Well, let's go, skinny! Hop on board!" the scale would say. It all felt so worth it. The scale and I were going to be buddies. Or better yet, more of a buddy/coach relationship. My resolve grew stronger. I needed to say no to all those temptations so I could receive my accolades every time I got on the scale in the morning. As I fell asleep after completing my first diet day (I was hungry, by the way), I couldn't wait to see how much weight I had lost the next morning. It kinda felt like Christmas Eve.

Weigh Out

I have a very specific ritual I follow before I weigh in:

1. Wake up and go to the restroom

2. Complete my workout, which at the time consisted of circuit training with weights and one hour of cardio on the treadmill

3. Revisit the restroom

4. Strip to my birthday suit

5. Hold on to the top of the shower stall as I ever so gently placed my weight one foot at a time on the scale (I didn't want to startle it)

6. Slowly let go of my grip on the shower stall to reveal my weight

7. Record the data

As I ever-so-smoothly placed my body onto my tried and true Health-O-Meter analog bathroom scale, I even held my breath so as to not jeopardize the accuracy of the scientific measurement I was in the process of taking.

Two hundred twenty-nine, 230, 231, 232, 233, 234, 235, 236, 237. Damn! I got off, moved the scale to a new position and measured myself again. Damn!

The second and third times were worse! I decided to record the first number, 237. My god, how could I be two pounds heavier!? I felt so deflated. "Maybe it's water weight," my wife suggested from behind me. "Or, you know, muscle weighs more than fat. Maybe that's it. Or I guess maybe the scale is broken." She was hoping to find anything to say that would make me feel better.

I clung to her last statement. "Maybe you're right. We've had this scale for a while; maybe it is broken. Here, you get on."

Then she backed away. "Hold on, buddy," she said, "I'm in a good mood. I'm not getting on that scale. It's never been nice to me. We are not on speaking terms, and that's just fine with me."

"Okay, okay," I said.

"Relax," she continued, "it's just your first day. Rome wasn't built in a day, right?"

"Yeah. You're right," I said. "Some experts say you shouldn't even weigh yourself for the first few weeks on a diet because it isn't accurate," she suggested.

"No," I said, "I want daily. It's probably just water weight. I did drink a lot of water yesterday."

"Yeah! I'm sure that's it," LaTeace said. "Maybe don't drink so much water today. Because you know even too much of a good thing is bad for you."

My wife was full of quips that morning and time was ticking. I still had to repeat what I had gone through the day before and still find time to work, have fun, and enjoy my life. But somehow, it seemed like my life was on hold. I felt lousy. I showered, got dressed, and began my day.

Growing up, my mom used to tell me to never judge a book by its cover, that it was the content that mattered. I knew that was true, but I didn't want to be fat because of what I thought it told everyone about me. I'm undisciplined, irresponsible, lazy, unreliable, but most of all I was unlovable. Weight for me became a blanket of shame. I didn't go to the pool without a shirt on: not because I didn't want to get sunburned (a damn good reason, by the way) but more because I wasn't proud of my body. Why did I care so much about what others thought of me? Why was I letting my self-worth be determined by the size of my body? I didn't know. Today wasn't my best day, but I wasn't giving in. Winners never quit and quitters never win. Suddenly, my head was filled with catchy quotes designed to make me feel better; my kind little voice inside me was back, but not for long.

Dr. Jekyll and Mr. Hyde

I'm not exactly sure when I first realized that there were voices in my head. Please don't think I'm crazy; I know everybody has that little voice inside their head, too. But the reason I say "voices," plural, is because it seems my little voice has a split personality. Sometimes it's encouraging and sometimes it's flat-out mean.

In fact, sometimes the little voice inside my head says such mean things to me, I wonder why I allow it to stick around. I always assumed it was me in there talking to me. One of my favorite books (next to *The Giving Tree*) is a book I discovered a few years ago called *The Untethered Soul* by Michael A. Singer. In it, I learned that this little voice inside my head wasn't even me! Those thoughts, feelings, emotions, memories, experiences, and sensations were all part of a very sophisticated data-processing system that is designed to do two very specific things: (1) Survive and (2) Reproduce.

Whoever our programmer was (don't want to get into a religious debate; natural selection and the grand design are not mutually exclusive) clearly didn't design us to know the meaning of life or design us to be born content. In fact, it's quite the opposite. Our creative designer actually programmed us to be dissatisfied. I guess it makes sense; if we were never programmed to ever feel bored, why would we ever get out of bed? If everything we did brought us pure contentment, we would never try anything new. No, in fact, our designer knew that a 100 percent content person rarely gets anything done. People who smoke pot are very content, which may be the reason that we just found out that anyone who lights up more than four times a week has lower productivity. We were designed to be bored quickly, and when we stumbled upon happiness, if we tried to stay too long in Happyville, our brains were designed to quickly come up with a reason to leave. Happy was designed to decay into sad. It's what keeps us alive.

Michael Singer points out in his book that we must not be the voices in our head because we are keenly aware when our thoughts and urges pop up. That which is aware of anything cannot be the object it is aware of. For example, let's say I'm looking at an apple. Obviously, I can't be the thing I'm looking at; I am the thing that is aware of the thing I am looking at. Even if I look in the mirror and see my reflection, I am not my reflection because my reflection is just light that bounced off me. Michael Singer explains it much more eloquently, but suffice it to say *we are not that which we are aware of; we are awareness itself.* You might need to let that sink in a little before you read on. It's important. Say it again if you have to. Okay, stay with me.

I have noticed since I was a tiny little child that sometimes I had thoughts that were nice to me and sometimes I had thoughts that were mean to me and they are grounded into two basic rules that govern us: (1) Survive and (2) Reproduce. This is just a spin-off of the first rule if we want our species to continue.

When we start tinkering around with food, we run smack into these two basic tenants of survive and reproduce. Our bodies use desires to drive us. When we are in Fear Mode, survive usually kicks in and when we are in Love Mode, reproduce takes over. Fear/Hate, Love/Desire are hardwired into us. It's like Dr. Jekyll and Mr. Hyde. Being on this diet was silencing poor kind Dr. Jekyll and releasing the evil Mr. Hyde. Fear had taken over my diet and Mr. Hyde was the voice in my head. And slowly but surely I was becoming someone nobody wanted to be around.

Thirty Days and Beyond

While the first thirty days were a walk on the darkside, I slowly managed to lose my first 11.3 pounds. With almost forty pounds to go, I can tell you that I felt what I imagined boot camp would be like. Every second of my life was regimented; from the time I woke up, I had meals at precisely the same time and sadly had a pretty unvaried meal plan. The romance of food was gone and had been replaced with scales and teaspoons and measuring cups.

I was winning the Battle of the Bulge, but was I losing the war? We were born with five senses; was being thin worth losing the sense of sight, touch, smell, and taste? If food wasn't to be savored, why did four of out five senses have to be sidelined? I knew I was choosing boring, tasteless food and could very well have chosen to put in the time and effort to make low-calorie tasty food, but when a meal is limited to 500 calories, how creative could I be? I can't tell you how torn I was. I missed having a vanilla shake with my Chick-Fil-A. I missed having French fries. I missed so much! I was thinner but I don't know how much happier. Every day was a roller coaster. My mood was tied to what the scale told me, and there didn't seem to be any rhyme or reason why one day I was three pounds heavier and the next down five. I didn't understand the huge fluctuations, but I did what I always do: I stuck with it.

When all the ups and downs were averaged out, I was truly losing weight. That felt good. It is nice to set a goal, especially a goal that literally holds your life in the balance, and achieve what you set out to do. The light at the end of the tunnel for me was 100 percent "good food" for me now, so I could mix some "good food" and "evil food" together once my prediabetic weight came down. I wasn't saying good-bye to all my mom's home-cooked recipes, it was more of a see ya later. That's what got me through the first thirty days and would eventually get me through the next six months. I would get to love food again later for turning my back on it now.

Looking back at the seven months it took to lose fifty pounds, I can honestly say it was one of the hardest things I had ever had to do. That and trying to pass a kidney stone. Those are my top two nightmares that still haunt me to this day. But once all the compliments came in, the shopping for new clothes, the feeling of success, it was easy to imagine that all those tasteless meals were somehow worth all the trouble. I had my health back, my blood pressure was down, and I did feel better. I certainly had a lot more energy! LaTeace and I decided to do some more traveling—Paris, London, Greece. The world was our oyster and now that I had a new body I was going to enjoy it.

The funny thing is, I didn't get to enjoy it for long. While I never allowed all the weight to come back, it was sneaking up on me. An extra pound of fat applied liberally to my body at Thanksgiving, another half pound at Christmas, and the ever-indulgent birthdays and anniversaries all started pushing my weight a little bit more each day. The day I hit 185 pounds was also the last day I would ever see that weight for a long time. I gave myself ten pounds of wiggle room between 185 and 195 and promised myself that the second I weighed over 195 I'd go back 100 percent on the diet from hell. "No pain, no gain" I've always been told. Nobody told me the game I was playing with my weight was a fixed game, where fat always makes a comeback and one where the player never wins.

CHAPTER 5

The Revenge of the
Body Snatchers

F or over ten years I kept that promise to myself. For ten years, I kept to my word that the second I went over 195 I would go on Def Con 1 and switch back to Hell Diet, and for ten years it worked—right up until the time it didn't.

October 24, 2014

The last few months had been very difficult; in July, we found out that my father-in-law was diagnosed with Stage 4 kidney cancer that had spread to his bones. It has a 95 percent mortality rate of five years. An atomic bomb had been dropped on our lives. So, it was no surprise that the time between hearing the news and stepping on the scale seemed like a blur.

When tragedy strikes it's hard to remember the commitments you've made to yourself and others. When your world implodes, the only thing you want to do is curl up into a ball and hide and my *modus operandi* was to curl up into a ball with comfort foods. Tom Hanks said in *A League of Their Own* that there is no crying in baseball. Well, I can attest that there is no crying in ice cream. Ice cream and I would see this through. It had been over three months since my foot had graced a scale and I can tell you I was more than a little scared. Already my clothes were fitting tight and my wife convinced me that stretch denim was my friend, not my enemy. I didn't want to get on the scale but I knew I had to face the music. I took a deep breath and stepped on. The kind little voice in my head said, "Don't worry; no matter how bad it is, we know how to solve it. Even if it's really bad news, the *Men's Health* diet will save us. The only problem to worry about is the one that has no solution."

Two hundred and ten. I weighed 210 pounds. No! I was fifteen pounds over my max! My heart started pounding. I felt a little faint and stepped off the scale. My eyes watered up. *It's not fair!* I said to myself. *I've been so good. I don't want to have to go on a strict diet again! I'm dealing with a dying father-in-law. It's just not fair!*

I had a flashback to a father and son talk in 1976. "What's the matter, son?"

"It's not fair, Dad! I get up every morning at four a.m. to practice basketball. I practice every second after school. I shoot over one thousand free throws a day. Why didn't I make the basketball team?!" I said and started to cry.

My dad put his arm around me and said, "I love you, son, and I am proud of you. What matters most is that you did your best."

"Well, apparently, my best isn't good enough," I said.

"Maybe this time it wasn't," he replied simply.

"That's not fair!" I cried.

"Son, I want to tell you something and I want you to never forget it. Come on, lift your head and look at me," my dad said. I wiped my eyes and nose and looked at my dad. He looked me straight in the eyes and said, "I don't know how to break it to you, but life isn't fair. But because it is equally unfair to everyone, that makes it fair."

I was confused and said, "I don't understand."

"That's okay. Someday you will," he assured me.

Flash forward. Was it fair that my father-in-law was dying from cancer? Was it fair that my mom had lost her eyesight to retinal degeneration? No, but since everyone must deal with unfairness, that makes it fair. I was fifteen pounds overweight and I wouldn't trade my problem for anyone else's. Cancer? Loss of sight? I was lucky to be fifteen pounds overweight.

Groundhog Day

My action plan was the same as before: STOP ALL EVIL FOOD and switch back to the *Men's Health* diet. I cleaned out my pantry, went shopping for groceries, and jumped right in. At the end of my first week I had gained 0.4 pounds and by the end of my second week I had gained another half a pound. This was debilitating. Two weeks and almost a full pound of weight gain. But I had seen this before; I know weight fluctuates greatly. I could have actually lost a pound or two and be holding on to three pounds of water. I was upset but not worried; by the end of the first month the highs and lows would balance out.

By the end of the first month, I was 1.7 pounds heavier than when I started. I was mentally, morally, and physically exhausted. This wasn't the same as before. Every day bad results. Every day the same thing. I reached out to the folks at *Men's Health* for some advice. Fortunately for me, we had worked on an article together back in December 2002, so I asked them to help me understand what I could possibly be doing wrong. I was referred to a recently published article by Michael Mejia. His advice was straightforward; I needed to change my training approach.

His article covered five key points:

1. *Identify Weaknesses*—look at my whole routine and find where my sticking point was. Where in my daily routine was I decelerating? If I could pick up my speed where I am normally slowing down, I could get over the hump. Sound advice!

2. *Think Small*—I may be trying to accomplish too much in my workouts or overdoing it in my calorie intake. If my body panics, I wouldn't lose weight. I needed baby steps. Got it! Dial it down.

3. *Do More*—While I may be thinking small, as in not overloading any one station of my life, I needed to increase my reps. If I do a lot of small

things right, it will lead to a big success. Once again, this made perfect sense.

4. *Lift Light*—On my off days, lighten my workload by 25 percent to allow the small blood vessels called capillaries in my body to recover. This will allow the essential oxygen, amino acids, and hormones to be delivered through my body so I can start dropping those pounds and building muscle.

5. *Move Faster*—Pick up my pace. Even a slight adjustment in my speed could kick start my metabolism. Boom! Great advice. Will do!

At the end of my second month I finally saw some progress. It was Christmas Eve and I had lost 0.2 pounds for the month. It had been two months and all I had to show for it was a 1½-pound weight gain. The only thing I could think was at least I was moving in the right direction. I was down 0.2 pounds in the toughest month of the year, December. I took my small victory. My guess was that by the end of January, I'd probably be seeing big gains.

By the end of January, I finally had something to smile about! I was down 1.7 pounds. Two months in a row with weight loss! While the mean voice in my head kept calling me a loser for only having lost 0.2 pounds for three months, I ignored all the taunts and forged ahead. This was moving at a snail's pace, but at least I had stopped gaining weight and the weight was coming off.

Breaking Point

In February 2015, I only had one cheat day and that was to celebrate my wife's birthday. I'll admit, the scale showed the weight instantly, but I was still shocked overall. I had gained four pounds in February!

For anyone who has ever been on a diet, you know what I was going through. I questioned everything! I beat myself up for splurging on my wife's birthday; I beat myself up for maybe not drinking enough water or getting enough sleep. Quite honestly, the kind little voice in my head hadn't visited me much anymore. This time around I had hit a brick wall and I didn't know what to do.

"If there's something strange in your neighborhood, who you gonna call? If there's something weird and it don't look good, who you gonna call? Gutbusters?" Nope. Google! Every time I have a problem that I couldn't solve, I googled it. I couldn't possibly be the only person on this planet with this problem; Google would supply the answer.

After trying out a few ways to frame "on diet, not losing weight," an article appeared right before my very eyes. It asked the question, "Are you someone with weight-loss resistance?" Hell yeah, I was! I read on. The article was by Marcelle Pick, OB/GYN NP. I wondered if the NP stood for No Problem. Just kidding; I knew it meant nurse practitioner. The article described everything I was going through to a T; following all the rules, eating just right, exercising, being a perfect student, yet no weight loss but gain! The article fit me exactly, except it was written for women. Okay, but the ideas presented here have got to cross over a little for men, too, so I kept on reading. Pick pointed to six areas that could be the cause of my weight loss failure.

They are:

1. Hormonal Imbalance (including thyroid dysfunction)
2. Adrenal Imbalance (chronic stress)
3. Neurotransmitter Imbalance
4. Digestive Imbalance
5. Systemic Inflammation
6. Impaired Detoxification

When I looked at the first letter of each cause, it spelled the word "HANDSI." I laughed. That would be easy to remember. *Okay,* I said to myself, *one or possibly all of these reasons are the cause of my weight-loss failure.* I spent the next three days studying each and every one so I could extract the true meaning of them. In the end, I could sum it all up in one sentence: if you are chronically scared or feel unsafe, your body will go into defense mode, circle the wagons, and hold on for dear life.

Huh. If I was fearful, I wouldn't lose weight. Was I scared? Hmm, maybe a little. But one thing became blatantly obvious: I needed to find a way to feel safe again, to somehow control my environment and not let it control me! I was the master of my destiny, not a slave to my circumstances! I was determined to double down on my commitment. I would hold on for dear life to get my weight and my life going in the right direction! I would never let go of control! I gave myself a mental high five. Hell, no! There is no quitter in me! The kind and loving voice was back in my head and it was cheering me on. "It doesn't matter if the house is on fire! Or that our world is in chaos! We got this! We can control this!"

I started to calm down and think of how silly it was that people couldn't lose weight just because they were a little fearful. Seriously, how silly is that? Everyone deals with the unknown. Everyone deals with fear. And fear? Forget about it! I was having none of it. I would take fear and push it further and further down so I didn't have to look at it. I control fear; it doesn't control me! I felt at peace, even if my stomach was all in knots. *Hold on*, I kept telling myself. I didn't realize that I was giving myself the very opposite advice I needed to hear.

I needed to **let go.**

Everything under Control

Starting in March 2015, I put my life under a microscope. Every conversation, every interaction, every moment was planned, calculated, executed, and documented. I had exact measurements for every calorie that went in my body and a calculation for every calorie burned through my workouts. I knew every calorie in and every calorie out. I would win this war!

At least that's what I thought until about two weeks into my new schedule when I woke up in the middle of the night with the most severe pain (next to having kidney stones) that I had ever experienced. Every attempt to swallow felt like I was swallowing razorblades. It was horrendous! I checked my temperature and it was over 102 degrees. My body was on fire. My body was quitting on me. My beautiful wife quickly got me to the doctor where I was diagnosed with strep throat. I was put on a prescription of antibiotics and antiseptic throat spray to numb the pain, and bedrest for at least seventy-two hours. But even with feeling I was on my deathbed, I dragged my body over to our home gym to work out each day. I would not be defeated on my hero's journey! Unbeknown to me, my immune system was shot and I was exacerbating the problem by not allowing my body to rest.

The three days turned into a week, but by the eighth day I did feel a little better. My temperature was gone and I was back on solid foods. The only side effect to my short stint of being sick was the absolute lethargy that had creeped into my body. I just felt completely exhausted.

After working out on that eighth day, assuming I just needed to recharge my batteries, I actually felt worse. When I looked in the mirror, I didn't recognize myself. I looked like a ghost with deep dark rings around my eyes and, in fact, one of my eyes was totally bloodshot! I blinked a couple of times and immediately knew what I had. Pink eye. I went to Google to see if pink eye was probable after having strep throat. Google told me yes. I took a picture of my eye, sent it to my doctor for confirmation, and was told yes, it was highly likely that I had pink eye. My eye would need steroids. I could not return to the office, because pink eye was highly contagious for at least another three days.

Why?! I said to myself. *Why is this happening to me!* Then I took a deep breath and said, *Everything will be okay. We got this under control. It's just a three-day delay.*

The second I put the first steroid drop into my eye it felt more like acid than a well-received bath. It burned so bad. The pain must mean it's killing the infection, I supposed. By the third day of treatment my eye looked worse and now my vision was blurry. My doctor no longer thought I had pink eye and sent me to my eye doctor, Doctor Sanders. It was there I was told I didn't have pink eye but herpes simplex keratitis. It was an infection of the cornea caused by the herpes simplex virus (HSV). If I didn't get treatment right away I ran the risk of losing my eye. Should I abandon my weight-loss goal? Should I abandon the commitments that I made to myself? No. I would keep my eye on the ball and save my eye at any cost.

Scarcity

When I was a little boy, my dad liked to tell me his life stories from growing up. Every one of them had a hidden life lesson if you paid close enough attention and looked for it. Of all the stories he told me, one of the ones that had the strongest impact on me was the Chicken Story.

The set up for the Chicken Story was always the same. My mom would have prepared a wonderful home-cooked meal. There were just the four of us—my sister, Mom, Dad, and I—but my mom always cooked as if she were feeding an army; no one went hungry in our home. My dad would lean back in his chair after we had said grace and dug into our food. He would say, "Slow down. The food isn't going anywhere. Your mom has cooked enough for seconds and leftovers. Enjoy."

My dad was and still is one of the slowest eaters I've ever seen. I've never met anyone who savors every bite like he does. While the rest of us were scarfing down our food and my mom was serving seconds, my dad just sat there taking his time; the world could just wait as he ate his meal. But eventually, sometime between our first and second serving, my dad would remind us how lucky we were to have such a bounty of food and that wasn't the way it always was in the Cuellar home.

There was a time when money and extras were stretched tight! I present to you now my father's chicken story . . .

"When I was your age living with your grandparents, things weren't as cushy as they are for you two and this family. I remember when it was chicken dinner night; of course there was your Uncle Alfonso, my brother, your Aunt Delia and Aunt Laura, my sisters, and, of course, your grandfather and grandmother, and me. But there was only the one chicken to feed the six of us. Your grandfather went first; he always chose a breast. Then my mom; she chose a breast. Then we'd each get a chance to pick the one piece we were allowed to have on this round. Naturally, the thighs and drumsticks always went in the opening round and then for the second round my parents would allow us each to have a second piece.

"Since there wasn't enough for everyone to have a second piece, my folks would bow out. What remained of the chicken was two wings, the back, and the neck. While the rest of us battled for the wings and back, your Aunt Laura always chose the neck, the one piece no one wanted. When I asked her why she chose the neck she said she needed to have something in her life she could count on, even if it was just the neck of a chicken.

"Every week when we knew which night was chicken night, your Aunt Laura needed to know what she was going to get. People can handle only so much uncertainty in their life. Of course, on the bright side, we did get all the rice and beans we wanted. Anyway, you two (my sister and I) should count your blessings that you have enough, heck, more than enough to eat, because there were times in this family there wasn't always extra."

Lesson to be gleaned from this story? Food can be scarce. There may be a day when you won't have enough to eat. That scared me. That's why I always cleaned my plate. That's why my relationship with food was complicated. In our family, food wasn't just food; it became a reward for everything. If we had a celebration, we did it with food. And if we were ever not grateful for the food on our plate, my dad would tell us the Chicken Story.

Hedonic Treadmill

In 1971, psychologists Brickman and Campbell published an essay titled "Hedonic Relativism and Planning the Good Society." Their essay suggested that regardless of what happens to someone that their level of happiness stays about the same. Twenty years later, Michael Eysenck, a British psychologist, modified the concept calling it "hedonic treadmill theory." He compared the pursuit of happiness to a person on a treadmill who must keep moving to just stay at the same place. The theory implies a "Happiness Set Point" we revert to given enough time. In essence, long-term happiness is not dependent upon short-term events. It may be devastating to lose a loved one, lose your job, to see your marriage collapse, to get sick, but if the happiness set point is true (and it appears to be true in study after study) we shouldn't sweat life's disappointments and pitfalls because we will adapt; we will cope.

And I'm not talking about just enduring; I'm talking about thriving, thriving in the face of adversity and maybe even because of it. Remember the four words that will make a happy man sad but yet make a sad man happy? "This too shall pass." That's adaptation. And it's not just for negative things, it's for positive things, too. In case after case of studying lottery winners, after their initial excitement and joy, they all returned to their original happiness set point after the win. If you weren't happy before winning the lottery, you would return to your unhappiness after the lottery. Happiness and unhappiness, order and chaos, live in us all and we all have different ways to deal with victories and disappointments.

The one thing that stood out most as I read about the hedonic treadmill was that the exception to a person returning to their happiness set point was prison. Once a person became an inmate, a prisoner, their happiness set point dropped. It would not return until their release. Apparently if you change a person's entire world and not just throw bombs or accolades on it, their happiness set point goes down. Environment regulates behavior and, apparently, happiness set points.

On April 1, 2015, I celebrated my fifty-second birthday. I was fighting to keep my right eye (and I would) and I was still trying to lose weight. But, by my birthday, I had only managed to lose 0.1 pound. My body was caught in a time warp. My sleep patterns were interrupted. I was exhausted all the time but I pressed on.

These are my weight-loss numbers for the next seven months:

April: 0.4-pound gain

May: 1-pound gain

June: 1-pound gain

July: 2.9-pound loss

August: 1.3-pound gain

September: 1.1-pound loss

October: 1.9-pound gain

I was on a hedonic treadmill but this time it wasn't just my happiness that was taken hostage, it was my weight. I had hit a weight set point. Every loss was demolished by a gain and I was back to where I started. I was moving but not going anywhere. In twelve months of a grueling, suffering diet I wound up six pounds heavier than I had started. My happiness set point had dropped and wouldn't bounce back up. It was as if my mind and body thought I was a prisoner of war. And actually, that's where I had allowed my thoughts to take me because I fought with my environment instead of embracing it. It wasn't until I realized that change wasn't my enemy that I would be allowed to see the light. And the light ended up being in the last place I expected; the light was in absolutely nothing at all.

CHAPTER 6

Cracking the Code

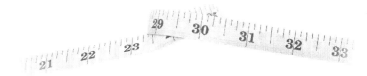

"He who has so little knowledge of human nature as to seek happiness by changing anything but his own disposition will waste his life in fruitless efforts."

— Samuel Johnson

n 1974, a professor of architecture and sculptor had an idea for a cube he could use to show his students a visual model of matter and how it could spin and move in space-time. The professor's name is Erno Rubik and his invention is the Rubik's Cube. In 1980 the Ideal toy company licensed his puzzle and began selling them. The cube was an instant sensation. Cube fever spread across the globe like wildfire; everyone wanted to get their hands on this multicolored, three-by-three-inch cube.

The premise was simple enough: the cube is solved when each face being one solid color; they are red, orange, yellow, green, blue, and white. The puzzle was in order, but with just a few twists and turns, the cube would take on over 43 quintillion combinations. That's 43×10^{18}, or 43 with 19 zeros after it. It's a lot of combinations! When the puzzle first came out, there were many who believed that unless you were a genius the cube was impossible to solve, and maybe there is some truth to that. The ability to think spatially and recognize patterns and develop an algorithm (a series of moves, a process, that if followed exactly will always give you the desired results) is hard.

I'll admit it, I was probably like the rest of you when you first played with the Rubik's Cube; I became interested, I became enthralled, I became exasperated, and then I quit. The cube was the first puzzle that I couldn't solve. After a while, Rubik's Cube solution books came out and for those willing to put the time in and learn the process, you, too, could solve the Puzzle of the Century! The funny thing was, even if you got your hands on the instruction manual, it was still kinda hard! There was a new language you had to learn and you had to learn how to hold the cube correctly. Even with the answer staring you dead in the face, it was still anything but easy.

In today's world, we call anything that is difficult or hard a "Rubik's Cube." Global warming is a Rubik's Cube. So is world peace. Weight loss is a Rubik's Cube.

I'm sure if you counted, there are probably more ways to try to solve the obesity problem on our planet than there are combinations to a Rubik's Cube. No matter how hard I tried, how many twists and turns I made, I was still a mess. The problem? Well, it wasn't that there weren't enough solutions being peddled, it was the fact that there wasn't any one solution that always worked. A *true* algorithm doesn't just work sometimes. It works all the time. Two plus two always equals four. If it didn't, we'd have a problem. We would be unable to write $X + X = 2X$. Substitute any number for "X" and the equation always balances out. The problem with all the "solution" books is you could insert one person in for X and the equation would balance but on other occasions it wouldn't. Was weight loss worse than a Rubik's Cube? Was weight loss an impossible cube, more like an egg dropped on the floor? One, that once the egg is broken, all the algorithms and solution books in the world couldn't put Humpty back together again?

Well, that's what I believed. I gave my diet twelve months of my life and had a six-pound gain to show for it. So you know what I did? I quit. Just like with the Rubik's Cube, I finally reached my breaking point. I had enough so I just gave up. With that one small decision of giving up, letting go, my chaotic world spun itself back into perfect order.

The Toyota Weigh

While many in my audience might think that I felt bad about quitting my diet, they would be incorrect. I was ecstatic! For the first time in a long time I felt I could breathe. If weight loss hadn't worked for many people, maybe it wouldn't work for me. Maybe I could be healthy fat? I still planned on working out, limiting my sweets, making healthy choices as often as I could; it's just that I refused to let food run my life anymore. I was back in charge! If I ended up being considered overweight on some "health chart," so what! My brain was coming up with one good reason after another for quitting my diet. I was happy for the first time in over a year and a half. One question that popped in my head was *What am I going to do with my newfound freedom? Hmm,* I thought to myself, *where would I focus my time?* Ah ha! Answer! I knew I wanted to brush up on my economics so I could be ready for some upcoming consulting work, so that's what I would do. Time for a good read!

Within thirty minutes, I downloaded the book, *The Goal: A Process of Ongoing Improvement (Thirtieth Anniversary Edition)* by Eliyahu M. Goldratt and Jeff Cox. It sold over six million copies and was considered the bible on the theory of constraints and how America does business. A business novel on how to run a successful supply chain was exactly what I was looking for.

Right from the beginning the author explains that the Goal was about science and education; science is the simplest way possible to derive a minimum set of assumptions that can explain a given phenomenon of nature, and education is a balance of reason and logical analysis of available facts.

Wonderful! This book was going to teach me how to use science and education to understand my world. I was ready to become smarter! I dug deeper. It didn't take me long to realize that the author was using the Toyota Production System (TPS) as a vehicle to help the main character solve the crises in his life. It is a famous method for aligning and running a lean assembly line for optimal utility. TPS was developed by Japanese industrial engineers Taiichi, Ohno, and Eiji Toyoda. It was the precursor to what is now generally referred to as "lean manufacturing" or "just-in-time production."

What these geniuses figured out was, quite simply, that where there is waste, there is chaos. And where there was chaos, there was a system that wasn't running efficiently. They identified three main categories of waste:

1. *Muda*—Nonvalue-adding work

2. *Muri*—Overburden

3. *Mura*—Unevenness

They then went on to describe the Seven Deadly Sins of Waste. They are as follows:

1. *Transport*—Anything that takes too long to go from point A to point B was a waste.

2. *Inventory*—Excess inventory that did not match demand raised operational costs and jeopardized the system. Beware of excess inventory!

3. *Motion*—Any action that did not benefit the process and created lag time must be eliminated. Don't waste energy.

4. *Waiting*—Between every action there can be unplanned delays. If the delays get out of hand, the system will bottleneck. A chain is only as strong as its weakest link.

5. *Overproduction*—Overproduction leads to excess inventory. It is important to not let

local efficiencies at workstations overproduce any product there wasn't a direct demand for. Overproduction leads to excess inventories, excess inventories lead to higher operating costs, and higher operating costs lead to death of the system. Hmm, this is a big one.

6. *Over-processed*—K.I.S.S.—Keep It Simple, Stupid! Don't overcomplicate anything or you'll create a traffic jam. "Simplicity, simplicity, simplicity," like Henry Thoreau said.

7. *Defects*—Recognize that it is impossible to make any large number of products without a percentage of them incurring defects. There needs to be allotted time to identify and repair defective parts.

The acronym derived from the above business model is TIM WOOD. The saying goes, "Don't be Tim Wood, not if you want to function efficiently." And then, like a stroke of lightning, it hit me: Oh my God! The human body is nothing more than an assembly line! And all at once, I began to cry.

Waste Away

Sitting right in front of me on a digital page was the entire outline, the entire framework for why diets work or don't work. It was plain as day. I quickly grabbed a notepad and pen and started writing feverishly. *Muda* was Japanese for "waste." If there was waste present in a system, the system would shut down. *Muri* was "stress" or "overburden" on the system. *Mura* was waste present in the system due to "unevenness," "inconsistency," or "randomness." *Muda, Muri, and Mura* were the environmental factors that would allow or disallow a system to function properly. And by system, I mean the human body.

Muda was the biggest, all-encompassing one. It represented the environment in which we placed our bodies. It was our home. It was our work; it was anywhere we spent a fair amount of time. If our environments that we lived in were cluttered, our lives would be cluttered; cluttered lives are not only chaotic, but stressful. If there was one thing I was quickly figuring out was that stress/fear locked up our bodies. When we were stressed out, we didn't lose weight. My God! It was obvious to me now: all those diets that exist in the world, most of them have sound science behind them, but they didn't get to the root cause of why we gain weight in the first place: *if we are stressed out, over-burdened, and have too much unpredictability, we can't lose weight.*

In fact, the opposite is true: basic thermal dynamics tells us that if you want something to have more energy/mass, just heat it up! If your environment is making you angry, heating you up, your body will absorb all that stress because at the end of the day, stress is a form of energy. If you are adding energy to your body, there is no reason you should weigh less, you should weigh more!

Okay. Step 1 was clear as day to me. It would be impossible for me to lose weight if my environment wasn't in order. I needed to remove all the nonessential things from the environments I lived in. My home seemed like the most logical place to start. But wait: how does one declutter one's life? I thought there had to be a book on it, so I went to Amazon and searched "How to declutter your life," The top search result stopped me in my tracks.

It was a book by Marie Kondo called *The Life-Changing Magic of Tidying Up: The Japanese Art of Decluttering and Organizing.* I was definitely on the right track. Within minutes by the magic of the cloud the book was in my iPad and I was reading through the table of contents.

Chapter 1: Why Can't I Keep My House in Order?

- You can't tidy if you've never learned how
- A tidying marathon doesn't cause rebound
- Tidy a little a day and you'll be tidying forever
- Why you should aim for perfection
- The moment you start you reset your life

Aha! That was it! I had stumbled upon another genius to help me on my Hero's Journey. Marie Kondo understood clearly that if we live in chaos our lives would be chaos and she turned to the Japanese for her insight, too! This couldn't be a coincidence! I ran home and told my wife we had to declutter our home if we wanted to change our lives. She immediately asked me to look around—did our home look like a mess? I had to admit that it didn't. My wife is a storage expert. Then I looked down at the sixth bullet point in chapter 1 "Storage experts are hoarders." I had a bigger problem than I thought.

Living in a Hoarder's Paradise

Scientists have long wondered what is going on in a hoarder's brain and fortunately now with brain scans the picture is starting to come into focus. Research published in the *Archives of General Psychology* done by David Tolin using functional magnetic resonance imaging (FMRI), 107 patients (43 with diagnosed hoarding disorder, 31 with OCD, and 33 with normal controls) were asked to bring a piece of their own junk mail or newspapers to the lab. The subjects were guaranteed none of their personal objects would be destroyed or discarded. While the participants had their brain scanned they were asked to think whether they should keep or shred the junk mail or newspaper. They were also shown junk mail that didn't belong to them and asked if it should be kept or shredded.

To no one's surprise, the hoarders chose to keep more things than those with OCD or control group. Michael Jenike, professor of psychiatry at Harvard, says, "Hoarders have great difficulty making decisions, especially around the value of their possessions." The hoarders' brains showed excessive activation in the anterior cingulate cortex; a brain region involved with decision making, especially in situations that involve conflicting information, doubt, or uncertainty. There was also elevated activity in the insula, the region of the brain that regulates one's emotional and physical state. It goes haywire in determining disgust, shame, anger, and all other negative emotions.

"This study is very interesting," says Michael Jenike, "as it demonstrates that brain regions associated with monitoring for errors under conditions of uncertainty are activated when hoarding patients are deciding whether or not to throw out personal items." Simply put: hoarders assign way too much value to their possessions, making it extremely difficult or impossible for them to decide to toss them out. Hoarders took much more time deciding about throwing anything out and felt a spiked anxiety and sadness even participating in the process. If the hoarder could convince himself or herself that there was some purpose for the item in the future, he or she could just not get rid of it, even if the likelihood of that purpose occurring was extremely remote.

What was even more surprising in the results was the hoarders made similar decisions to keep junk mail that didn't belong to them and felt the same discomfort even though the mail had nothing to do with them. Given enough time, hoarders could always come up with a plausible reason for keeping anything. The paper's authors noted that the hoarders' reactions were similar to patients with autism who are often disengaged from others and tend to follow rigid routines and act obsessively.

My wife's favorite saying since the day I met her has been, "It's better to have and not need than need and not have." At the time, it made perfect sense. Where would our lives be if we weren't prepared? Wasn't that the Boy Scout's motto? Be Prepared! But clearly, there was a line, a line if crossed where you could be over-prepared, where stuff became mountains and mountains became too high to climb. If we can justify holding onto the garbage in our lives, how could we ever get rid of excess fat? The short answer is we can't.

The question the hoarders were asking themselves turned out to be the wrong question. It wasn't, "Is there some possible use for this item in the future?" to which the answer is always yes. We can justify anything, for God's sake! No, the question should be, "Is this—garbage, relationship, stuff—that's in my life, is it making my life more or less convenient?" All that matters is the present moment; no one knows what the future holds. If the answer to that question was "less convenient" and taking too much of your time, it must go. If anything in our lives was gobbling up our valuable time and not giving us a return on our investment, it has to be let go!

By the time my wife and I got done decluttering our home, we had filled over eighty large, green garbage bags with junk. Once it was gone, we felt . . . well, free, like a weight had been taken off our shoulders. We were finally living in a Hoarder's Paradise, where everything we kept served us and not the other way around; we were out of our Hoarder's Hell. Einstein once said, "Nothing happens until something moves." Getting rid of all the nonessential things in our lives not only gave us room to breathe, it gave us the open space to grow.

Waste Not, Want Not

Once I cleaned up my environment (which was Step 1 to turning my life around), I had to move to Step 2, *Muri*—how did I manage my time? If time was everything, was I wasting my time? Efficiency does many things; effectiveness does only what needs to be done. Was I living an effective life or one where I was just chasing my tail and running around in circles going nowhere? I charted how I spent every hour of my time for an entire week.

Seven days a week, I woke up no later than 6:50 a.m. I worked out seven days a week, worked Monday through Friday, nine to five, and Saturdays nine to noon. I was off on Saturday afternoons and Sundays. When I got home from work, my iPad was always at my side until ten o'clock. I kept it there to quickly jot down notes, look up information, or write down any new ideas or to-dos. Hmm . . . time for my friends, family, vacations, social events, concerts, etc., wasn't there. I woke up, worked out, went to work, came home, ate, gave my wife my partial attention (because I was essentially still working in my head) until I went to bed between ten thirty and eleven o'clock. Work, sleep, and eat. I was chasing my tail; I was going nowhere. I was wasting my time, my life. I was overburdening myself with things that just didn't matter. It wasn't like my "to-do list" was ever really going to be completed. And did I really have to look at my emails and texts every two seconds? Technology was supposed to make my life better, but all these smart devices did was allow me to work more and live less. Of course I wasn't losing weight; my priorities were all wrong.

Muri is a Japanese word meaning "unreasonableness; impossible; beyond one's power." I was trying to make the world's problems my problems. I was trying to do forty-eight hours of work in a twenty-four-hour day. I was overburdening my life with task after task that in the big scheme of things didn't matter. I remember watching a documentary about the pursuit of happiness and the clinicians determined that there were two paths to try and find happiness.

One path followed extrinsic values: rewards (money), praise (the adulation of others), and status (stuff). Anyone who followed this path always ended up in a dead end. Happiness is not something that can be found outside of you.

The other path followed intrinsic values: personal growth, relationships, helping others. The people on this path didn't have to search for happiness; they carried it with them as a light that burned inside their soul, a light that not only enriched their lives but the lives of everyone they encountered.

No, sadly, I was on the path most traveled and I needed to make some changes before it was too late. I needed to tell the people in my life that I love them and that I am sorry for taking them for granted. I needed to unplug from the work grid and give the people and things I love my undivided attention. I needed to be of service, help those less fortunate than me, and make a difference in other people's lives.

The reality was, I had to realign my values and put love first and not "success" or money.

My dad once joked with me that the man who dies with the most toys wins. I know now that isn't correct. The man who dies with the fewest "things" and strongest relationships is the one who wins. *Muri* allowed me to realize where I was wasting my time, allowing myself to be overburdened by things that, in the end, don't really matter. I wasn't born to make money or just survive. I was born to love and be loved. That would lead to my new mantra: "To the degree you love, you will be loved." Why love others? Because as the Beatles said, "All you need is love."

Balance

Once upon a time, a long, long time ago, there was a kingdom called the United States of America. In this kingdom lived a king (president) named Abraham Lincoln. Abraham Lincoln believed in a concept called "equality for all." Many people in the kingdom didn't like what he stood for and eventually there was a huge battle over this one simple idea. Between 1861 and

1865, opposing sides fought for their definition of justice. Was equality and freedom for some or was it for all?

As we all know, liberty for all won the day, civil rights were guaranteed, Reconstruction began, and attempts to restore unity to the kingdom began. But it wasn't until two months after the death of Abraham Lincoln on April 15, 1865, that the last shot was fired in the Civil War on June 22. A man died for equality. A kingdom was torn apart and had to be stitched back together. But was there equality? Not hardly. The mentality of slavery doesn't go away overnight. Slavery can live in a man's heart long after laws are passed that ensure his freedom, and if slavery lives in the heart of any man, it lives in the kingdom of all men.

On August 20, 1866, a new organization named the National Labor Union asked Congress to pass a law mandating the eight-hour workday. Their efforts failed. Twenty-four years later the U.S. government began tracking workers' hours. The average workweek for full-time employees was an astounding one hundred hours! The average life expectancy of those workers was forty-five years of age. Was working yourself to death freedom? It wasn't until June 25, 1938, that Congress passed the Fair Labor Standards Act, which limited the workweek to forty-four hours. By June 26, 1940, it was amended to a forty-hour workweek.

The third head of the serpent of waste is *Mura*. *Mura* is Japanese for "unevenness," "irregularity," "lack of uniformity," or "inequality." Where there is inequality, there is waste. I had to bring equality to my life if I was going to ever get my health back. I spent an average of 105 hours of my week, fifteen hours of my day, thinking or participating in work. The rest of my day I was too exhausted to do anything else. Where was the equality?

It didn't exist. I was master of my life but a slave to myself. I was working to death. My body had been trying to tell me with the weight gain that it needed a break, but I hadn't been listening.

There are three main areas in our lives that must be even or our lives will be out of balance. They are: our work life, our personal life (those are the hours that just belong to us), and our maintenance life (the hours we spend maintaining the relationships and things we value most). There was no evenness or equality in any of those three areas of my life. If I was going to eliminate *Mura* and restore balance to my life, I would have to work less, rest more, and maintain the relationships in my life better. I had to shift time, not make time, from where I was overburdened to where I was starving.

On November 1, 2015, I enacted the forty-hour workweek in my life, and with it freed myself to sleep, read, learn, grow, and spend time with my loved ones. My emancipation proclamation declared I would spend my time evenly among work, self, and relationships. The original Emancipation Proclamation was passed in 1863. One hundred years later, in 1963, I was born. And now, fifty years after that, I was finally free.

When Decay Stops, Growth Begins...

Muda, Muri, and *Mura* were the three environmental factors that were destroying my life. I had allowed myself to live in a cluttered, overburdened, and unbalanced world. It was nobody's fault but mine. I was asleep at the wheel of my own life.

In 1946, Viktor Frankl published *Man's Search for Meaning.* Viktor Frankl was a Holocaust survivor; he lost all of his family members, including his wife, in concentration camps. They were murdered. Most people describe what happened to those who lost their lives in concentration camps as being "exterminated." I find the use of the word grotesque—which, perhaps it is supposed to be. We exterminate bugs, not people.

It is estimated that over eleven million lives were lost during the Holocaust. The word *holocaust* means "destruction or slaughter on a mass scale." Historically, it meant a Jewish sacrificial offering that is burned completely on an altar. Viktor Frankl survived that. I think it is fair to say that if any one of us lost all of our loved ones and witnessed an extinction of eleven million people, we might be a little bitter. We might be a little angry. We might even hold on to that anger until we, too, were buried alongside our loved ones.

But that's not what Frankl did. He rose above it and said probably the most elegant thing I have ever read or have heard in my life: "It is not the load we carry but how we choose to carry the load that matters."

If those words don't take you back, nothing will. Frankl was trying to tell us that regardless of our circumstances, regardless of our suffering, how bad or good the hand we're dealt, we can rise above it. We can derive any meaning of anything that happens to us in our lives. If we wanted to be a victim, it was our choice. The victor? Our choice, too. We and only we can tell the story of our lives. And it's not found in the facts of our lives but how we choose to define the expected and unexpected events that occur. Like my dad said, "Life is unfair, but because it is unfair to everyone makes it fair." Regardless of your environment, you can either change it or leave it, but you are not powerless. The meaning of our lives is all in how we choose to interpret anything.

Muda, Muri, and *Mura* all say the same thing: *don't waste your time.* Time is the most precious commodity you'll ever own. The seven subtypes of waste according to Lean Manufacturing are:

1. Transport
2. Inventory
3. Motion
4. Waiting
5. Overproducing
6. Over-processing
7. Defects

Why did they have to be seen as waste? That's not what I saw when I learned those categories; I saw the Seven Ways to Being Healthy. These were the seven questions I wrote down when I finally figured out why my life was going nowhere:

1. *How is fuel for the body transported?*
2. *How is inventory made for the body?*
3. *How does motion affect my body?*
4. *How can waiting to eat work for me?*
5. *How can I stop overproduction of fat?*
6. *How can I deal with over-processed food?*

7. *How do I make desire for food work for me instead
   of against me?*

I laughed; I already knew all the answers to the questions.
Now let me tell you . . .

CHAPTER 7

The Seven Healthy Questions

When I was young, it could easily be argued that I was hard-headed. If I believed anything enough, it would take heaven and Earth to get me to change my mind. This was especially true if I believed something negative. Once I had a negative opinion about anything, it was very difficult for me to change my mind.

One of the negative beliefs I had was that I wasn't as smart as others. This dysfunctional belief came out of the observation that it appeared to me that it took me longer in school to get whatever new idea or concept the teacher was trying to get us to understand. If a teacher said, A + B = C, my hand immediately went up.

"What is 'A'?" I would ask, to which the teacher would respond, "It can be any number." And I would say, "That doesn't make sense, obviously, 'A' can't be any number because if 'A' were any number that would include the number 'B' and 'C'. And if that were the case, the equation would be A + A = 2A."

"Please sit down and be quiet, Mr. Cuellar! No one likes your antics."

She thought I was playing but I wasn't. Every time I was told a so-called fact, my mind would fill with a myriad of questions that I needed an answer to before I would just blindly accept what was being fed to me. For that, I got punished. My conclusion was, "Everyone else gets what's being taught and I don't. I must not be as smart as everyone else." I had and still have to know everything about a subject before my brain will relax and say, "Yeah, okay, that makes sense. I get it." Understanding why the human body responded how it did to weight gain was no exception.

To the rest of the world, it was simple: you gain weight when you eat too much and don't exercise enough. I had proven to myself that it wasn't that simple; it was much more of a puzzle than that. But a puzzle that once you got it, like the algorithm to the Rubik's Cube, you'd never forget it. Kinda like a safe lock that's been closed right up until the combination is put into motion and all the tumblers fall into place and the door swings open.

"Why man couldn't maintain his weight" was solved in my mind and it all stemmed from the answers to the "Seven Questions for Growth" I stated at the end of Chapter 6. The funny thing was once I got the solution, it suddenly seemed so obvious to me that I didn't understand why I or anyone else hadn't solved the puzzle before. My dad always told me growing up that when I was an adult, life would be much more difficult. As a child you're always given the questions that you have to find the answers to, but as an adult no one tells you what the questions are; you have to figure them out. Well, it had taken me years but I finally knew what the questions were. Let's go over the answers. It's time for you to be healthy.

1. How is fuel for your body transported?

I'd like for you to imagine for just a second that all the veins in your body are like roads and highways. The blood that travels through your veins is like cars, busses, and trucks. The passengers, the cargo, are food. To make this analogy even simpler, I want you to picture an elementary school packed with kids all bustling around going from class to class; a bundle of energy. We will say that there are three kinds of kids in the school: the Proteins, the Fats, and the Carbs. If we associated endurance with caloric value, the Fats would be the most powerful with nine calories per gram, followed by the Proteins and Carbs coming in tied for second at four calories per gram.

When the school day ends and the final bell rings, all the kids go rushing to the waiting school busses outside to take all the kids home (the organs of our bodies). After all the busses are loaded, some packed (standing room only), some partially full and some totally empty, the busses head out for their routes. Not all the kids got on the busses because each bus represents a meal that was consumed or skipped. Skipped school busses leave the school with no kids on board. Of course, the partial school busses we could easily describe as snack meal busses; they only have a few students and won't necessarily be able to make it to all the stops. Rarely is a school bus perfectly balanced, usually the busses leave the school partially empty or stuffed. All the busses spend two-and-a-half to five hours max in traffic (the stomach) as each kid changes from his school uniform to his play clothes. The kids can't do what they want to do if they aren't allowed to play. The Fats change into Fatty Acids, the Proteins change into Amino Acids, and the Carbs turn into Glucose.

After they are through the traffic jam, the busses turn off to a long and winding road called the small intestine. It is there that all the kids are dropped off and sent on their way to play and energize their homes (our organs). The Carbs are always first off the bus and always hit the ground running; they are like sprinters who are good at the hundred-yard dash but are lousy distance runners.

The next off the bus are the Proteins; they have a little more stamina and can play longer than the Carbs. They aren't quite the distance runners of the Fats, but they make good time on the mile. For eight hours, all the kids jump off the bus and find their homes—that is except when the homes are full.

Your organs can only handle so many rowdy kids, and once they've had their fill, any extra kids that over-packed the school busses are forced to go to orphanages. The orphanages are holding cells that lie in our liver, muscles, and under our skin in fat cells. Fat cells are Motel 6s that always have occupancy. They never turn any kids away. The kids in the orphanages are not allowed to play and are forced to keep their energy until they get to one day go to an organ in the body as fuel. But for now, they are fuel storage.

The Carbs that changed into glucose are changed again into their pajamas and stored as glycogen. The Proteins and Fats that changed into Amino Acids and Fatty Acids to play are also changed again into their pajamas for a long slumber as they become triglycerides (what we know as fat).

After five hours in the stomach, and three hours in the gut or small intestine, the empty buses head back to the large intestine (end of the line) after all the nutrition has been squeezed out of them, either in the form of energy (play) or stored energy (fat). All the kids end up somewhere; no child is left behind. The thing is, nowadays most kids never get to play; they are forced to live as potential that is never realized because someone didn't know how to pack the bus.

2. How is inventory made for the body?

Before we can go into detail of how inventory is made in the human body, let's first define what inventory is. Inventory is any fuel that is made by the consumption of fats, proteins, and carbs that there is not a current demand for. By definition, inventory is a reserve; a backup supply that the body keeps for emergencies. If your body didn't keep a reserve inventory of fuel you would run the risk of your body self-cannibalizing if there was ever a fuel (food) shortage.

While it may appear self-evident that any person who eats more than their body needs will create inventory either in glycogen reserves stored in the liver and muscles or triglyceride reserves stored around the body in the form of fat, this still begs the question: What does a body need, besides, of course, good loving? Well, that's different from person to person, even from male to female. While there are a ton of formulas to figure out how much fuel (calories) a body needs, my favorite is the Hamwi Equation. In 1964, Dr. G. J. Hamwi developed formulas to help calculate ideal weights for men and women. They originally appeared in a publication of the American Diabetes Association. They are very straightforward.

Hamwi Equation for a Woman

A woman should weigh one hundred pounds for her first five feet of height and an additional five pounds for every inch after that. *Example:* a five-foot-four woman should ideally weigh 120 pounds. One hundred pounds for the first five feet and twenty pounds for the additional four inches.

Since men tend to have more muscle mass than women, the equation is different.

Hamwi Equation for a Man

A man should weigh 106 pounds for his first five feet of height and an additional six pounds for every inch after that. *Example:* A man who is six feet tall should ideally weigh 178 pounds; one hundred and six for the first five feet and an additional seventy-two pounds for the extra twelve inches.

Keep in mind that these are generalizations and guidelines. Obviously if you pump iron every day and you have more lean muscle mass, there could be up to 20 percent variance. Quite a few people use a Body Mass Index (BMI) chart (see next page) to see what healthy ranges are. We need to have some body fat (inventory) but the key here is we don't want excess inventory.

Body Mass Index (BMI) Chart for Adults

Obese (>30) | Overweight (25-30) | Normal (18.5-25) | Underweight (<18.5)

Weight (lbs)	4'8"	4'9"	4'10"	4'11"	5'0"	5'1"	5'2"	5'3"	5'4"	5'5"	5'6"	5'7"	5'8"	5'9"	5'10"	5'11"	6'0"	6'1"	6'2"	6'3"	6'4"	6'5"
260	58	56	54	53	51	49	48	46	45	43	42	41	40	38	37	36	35	34	33	32	32	31
255	57	55	53	51	50	48	47	45	44	42	41	40	39	38	37	36	35	34	33	32	31	30
250	56	54	52	50	49	47	46	44	43	42	40	39	38	37	36	35	34	33	32	31	30	30
245	55	53	51	49	48	46	45	43	42	41	40	38	37	36	35	34	33	32	31	31	30	29
240	54	52	50	48	47	45	44	43	41	40	39	38	36	35	34	33	33	32	31	30	29	28
235	53	51	49	47	46	44	43	42	40	39	38	37	36	35	34	33	32	31	30	29	29	28
230	52	50	48	46	45	43	42	41	39	38	37	36	35	34	33	32	31	30	30	29	28	27
225	50	49	47	45	44	43	41	40	39	37	36	35	34	33	32	31	31	30	29	28	27	27
220	49	48	46	44	43	42	40	39	38	37	36	34	33	32	32	31	30	29	28	27	27	26
215	48	47	45	43	42	41	39	38	37	36	35	34	33	32	31	30	29	28	28	27	26	25
210	47	45	44	42	41	40	38	37	36	35	34	33	32	31	30	29	28	28	27	26	26	25
205	46	44	43	41	40	39	37	36	35	34	33	32	31	30	29	29	28	27	26	26	25	24
200	45	43	42	40	39	38	37	35	34	33	32	31	30	30	29	28	27	26	26	25	24	24
195	44	42	41	39	38	37	36	35	33	32	31	31	30	29	28	27	26	26	25	24	24	23
190	43	41	40	38	37	36	35	34	33	32	31	30	29	28	27	26	26	25	24	24	23	23
185	41	40	39	37	36	35	34	33	32	31	30	29	28	27	27	26	25	24	24	23	23	22
180	40	39	38	36	35	34	33	32	31	30	29	28	27	27	26	25	24	24	23	22	22	21
175	39	38	37	35	34	33	32	31	30	29	28	27	27	26	25	24	24	23	22	22	21	21
170	38	37	36	34	33	32	31	30	29	28	27	27	26	25	24	24	23	22	22	21	21	20
165	37	36	34	33	32	31	30	29	28	27	27	26	25	24	24	23	22	22	21	21	20	20
160	36	35	33	32	31	30	29	28	27	27	26	25	24	24	23	22	22	21	21	20	19	19
155	35	34	32	31	30	29	28	27	27	26	25	24	24	23	22	22	21	20	20	19	19	18
150	34	32	31	30	29	28	27	27	26	25	24	23	23	22	22	21	20	20	19	19	18	18
145	33	31	30	29	28	27	27	26	25	24	23	23	22	21	21	20	20	19	19	18	18	17
140	31	30	29	28	27	26	26	25	24	23	23	22	21	21	20	20	19	18	18	17	17	17
135	30	29	28	27	26	26	25	24	23	22	22	21	21	20	19	19	18	18	17	17	16	16
130	29	28	27	26	25	25	24	23	22	22	21	20	20	19	19	18	18	17	17	16	16	15
125	28	27	26	25	24	24	23	22	21	21	20	20	19	18	18	17	17	16	16	16	15	15
120	27	26	25	24	23	23	22	21	21	20	19	19	18	18	17	17	16	16	15	15	15	14
115	26	25	24	23	22	22	21	20	20	19	19	18	17	17	16	16	16	15	15	14	14	14
110	25	24	23	22	21	21	20	19	19	18	18	17	17	16	16	15	15	15	14	14	13	13
105	24	23	22	21	21	20	19	19	18	17	17	16	16	16	15	15	14	14	13	13	13	12
100	22	22	21	20	20	19	18	18	17	17	16	16	15	15	14	14	14	13	13	12	12	12
95	21	21	20	19	19	18	17	17	16	16	15	15	14	14	14	13	13	13	12	12	12	11
90	20	19	19	18	18	17	16	16	15	15	15	14	14	13	13	13	12	12	12	11	11	11
85	19	18	18	17	17	16	16	15	15	14	14	13	13	13	12	12	12	11	11	11	10	10
80	18	17	17	16	16	15	15	14	14	13	13	13	12	12	11	11	11	11	10	10	10	9

Height (in feet/inches)

*BMI values rounded to the nearest whole number.

So how do we accomplish that? How do we make sure we don't store excess inventory or fat? Well, once we've calculated what our body requires to function properly, it's a piece of cake! Ugh, now I'm thinking of cake. Just kidding.

Here's what you do: multiply your ideal weight by ten to determine your minimum energy requirement. For example, let's take the five-foot-four woman from before who ideally should weigh 120 pounds. We would take 120 × 10 and that would equal 1,200. What is the 1,200? It's calories. This woman requires at a minimum 1,200 calories to just exist. And by "just exist" I mean to just lay in bed and do nothing.

Earlier I mentioned something called a Basal Metabolic Rate, or BMR. Our BMR represents how many calories our bodies need just to maintain our existence. It takes energy to do everything your body requires, from breathing, thinking, and metabolizing food to running our organs. Even while you sleep your body is always gobbling up energy from your fuel tanks to keep you alive. Obviously, though, we do more than lay in bed all day (I'm assuming). Even a sedentary person needs 30 percent more calories than their BMR requires to navigate their day.

Here's how to figure out how many more calories you'll need depending on how active you are:

Extremely Active: BMR × 2

Active: BMR × 1.5

Sedentary: BMR × 1.3

Example: Back to the five-foot-four woman. She needs

- 1,200 to just lie in bed,
- 1,560 calories (1,200 × 1.3) to be sedentary,
- 1,800 calories (1,200 × 1.5) to be active, and
- 2,400 calories (1,200 × 2) to be extremely active.

If the goal is to maintain an ideal weight, then the caloric intake would have to fall within these brackets.

Interestingly, this isn't the whole picture. There are people in this world who can't sit still; I call them tappers. You know those folks: even while they're sitting, they tap their foot on the floor. These are fidgeters, and fidgeting burns calories. The official term is N.E.A.T. calories. N.E.A.T. stands for Non-Exercise Activity Thermogenesis. If you're always moving, it burns calories, even if it's not traditional exercise.

Back to the original question: How does inventory (fuel reserves) get made? By consuming more calories than are required for operating your ideal weight. Do this long enough and you and me and anyone else will stop being healthy, become overweight, and eventually obese. If inventories rise too high, operating expenses skyrocket. And if operating expenses get too high, well, the system fails. And you, my friend, are the system.

3. How does motion affect the body?

In 1687 Isaac Newton compiled the three laws of motion in his book *Philosophiae Naturalis Principia Mathematica* (*Mathematical Principles of Natural Philosophy*). Newton used the laws to help explain the motion of physical objects and systems. Why did something move? Why did something stop moving? Why did something never stop moving? Why did something never move? What was at the heart of motion? Did something move because an outside force moved it? Or was there a force deep within the system that gave itself the force to move? Or was it both; could an object at once be moved by outside forces and have the internal force to be swayed by that force and push back against it?

Let's examine each of the three laws and see how a man we've never met from 1687 and his laws can have such a profound effect on our lives today.

Newton's First Law

Bear with me. This is exactly what it says in Wikipedia about Newton's First Law. I will quote it verbatim and then put it in a language that the average Joe can understand. If you haven't figured it out by now, I like to present information in the easiest format possible. If a child can understand a concept, then so can anyone else. Here's the complicated explanation for Newton's First Law:

"The first law states that if the net force (the vector sum of all forces acting on an object) is zero, then the velocity of the object is constant. Velocity is a vector quantity which expresses both the object's speed and direction of motion; therefore, the statement that the object's velocity is constant is a statement that both its speed and direction of its motion are constant."

Interpretation for anyone to understand: if you don't mess with an object at rest, it will stay at rest. If you don't mess with an object in motion, it will stay in motion. Why do people move? Someone or something pushed them or they pushed themselves. It takes force, physical or mental, to get anything moving. And it takes physical or mental force to stop anything. There are four forces in the universe: Strong Force, Weak Force,

Electromagnetic, and Gravity. Without these forces, there would be no matter, no space, no way to relate anything. At zero degrees kelvin (absolute zero) there is no energy and no motion. And if there is no energy and no motion, there is no time. "Space" between things would not exist. We would not exist. It takes force to make us and it takes force to move or stop us. In essence, we are a force. When a force stops moving, it stops existing. Whether the first law intended to convey that meaning or not, it doesn't make that any less true. If our bodies (our force) stop moving or never stop moving, we cease to exist. Lesson? There is a time to move and there is a time to rest. We must do both.

Newton's Second Law

Technical Wikipedia description: "The vector sum of the forces, (F) on an object is equal to the mass (m) of that multiplied by the acceleration vector (a) of the object. $F = ma$."

We touched on that in Chapter 1. If we want to know how big or how small something is, just pay attention to how much it moves. Things that move very slowly or not at all tend to be bigger than things that can accelerate and move quickly. Lesson: If we pay attention to how quickly we can move, if we make time for moving, we can guide our bodies in the right direction. When anything loses its purpose, it tends to move less. Motion (physical) and emotion (mental) are the forces we use to not only stay alive but also to keep our mind-bodies healthy. No force, no movement, no matter.

Newton's Third Law

Wikipedia: "When one body exerts a force on a second body, the second body simultaneously exerts a force equal in magnitude and opposite in direction on the first body."

We get nothing back in this world other than what we put in. If you push the world it will push back. What we do or fail to do for others matters. What we do or fail to do for ourselves matters.

Why is motion important to the human body? Because without action nothing gets done. Our bodies stay at rest. There is no acceleration and we waste away. Three laws, one message: get moving and get living, or get dying.

4. How can waiting to eat work for me?

According to the U.S. Department of Agriculture, approximately 72 percent of men and 64 percent of women are classified as overweight or obese. As a nation, are we a country that's waiting to eat? No. The typical American is having fourteen to twenty-one meals a week (a meal is defined as any eating event over five-hundred calories) and anywhere from thirty-five to forty-nine "snacks" (eating event that puts any calories in your system under five-hundred calories per event). If you look at the top number, Americans are eating or drinking something with calories ten times a day. It appears that the second we believe we are hungry we search out food. So, where do beliefs of hunger come from? Can we trust ourselves when we believe we are hungry?

We will take the questions in order. *Cues trigger our belief of hunger more than anything else.* When we see or smell food our digestive system thinks we are going to eat and starts the digestive juices in our stomachs to get ready for the meal. The growling in your stomach rarely means you're actually hungry; it just means you've recently seen food (perhaps in a commercial, around the office, or at home) or smelled food. We also have formed a bad habit of associating certain times of the day with eating times. At noon, we figure we'd better eat lunch. By five or six, we figure we'd better get some dinner. Most of the time when we "think" we are hungry our bodies are just responding to environmental cues to eat. The reality is, true hunger or starvation can't happen in a few hours. A body doesn't begin to think it's starving until it has lost 30 percent of its body weight. Not many of us lose 30 percent of our body weight because we missed out on a meal or snack.

The second question: can we trust ourselves when we think we are hungry? Usually, no. The typical person gets a "it's time to eat" thought sixty to ninety minutes after any meal (even large meals over one-thousand calories). Do you really think your body needs food? No. As it turns out, sixty to ninety minutes after you've eaten, your digestive system sends a hormone to your brain called ghrelin. It's the hunger hormone. Your digestive system is asking your brain (your hypothalamus) if it's going to be sending any more food down, because if it isn't, it will wrap things up. Your body isn't saying it wants more food, it's just asking if you're done eating. If you think you're hungry, stop. Look at your watch. If it's been less than three hours since your last meal, you're not hungry. Don't eat. If you've had a full-tank, balanced meal (typically over one-thousand calories), your body technically won't need any food for ten hours (five hours maximum digestive time in the stomach, three hours for second press of nutrients in small intestines, two hours of rest time). But even after ten hours of no food you won't starve. Just about all of us have over 10 percent body fat (a typical American has over 30 percent body fat) and 10 percent body fat would keep you alive for thirty days, assuming you had water. Are we a country of starving people? Not hardly.

If not waiting to eat is causing the problem, then the answer to the obesity problem is simple: *we need to eat less often; fewer meals, not more. And the meals we do eat must be satisfying.* Since taste is what drives most of us to eat, if we are going to delay gratification we'd better make sure when we get a good meal it is something we really want. We're eating a lot of meals and snacks and we aren't even satisfied.

Waiting is a buffer, a zone where we declare we aren't eating. No snacks, no junk. We give our bodies an opportunity to process the last meal we had. Instant gratification is the key to obesity. Delayed gratification is the key to a healthy body. Our mind-set has to be "less meals that mean more to us." To grasp where I'm going with this, you have to know the following four laws of weight management.

The Four Laws of Weight Management

Law #1: SATISFACTION INCREASES: Calories go up per meal and frequency of meals goes down.

Law #2: SATISFACTION DECREASES: Calories go down per meal and frequency of meals goes up.

Law #3: BODY FAT INCREASES: Calories go down per meal and frequency of meals goes up.

Law #4: BODY FAT DECREASES: Calories go up per meal and frequency of meals goes down.

We are so used to hearing the same old tired advice: eat less, exercise more, have a lot of little meals throughout the day to keep your metabolism running high, count your calories, change the size of the plate you eat from, eat only half of the food on your plate, eat at restaurants less, avoid carbs, eat like a caveman, etc. No wonder we are overweight.

There are two things that make you hungry: eating and exercise. So, what do experts tell us to do? Eat more small meals and exercise like crazy to earn our meals. Ridiculous! Go out on a fishing boat and throw a little chum (bait consisting of fish parts, bone, and blood) into the water and watch all the fish that are attracted. It will cause a feeding frenzy! Every time we put even the smallest amount of food into our bodies, it's like throwing chum into the water. Our bodies want more! Eating makes you hungry up until the moment your stomach's volume sensors signal full. Then the hormone leptin is sent to the brain to tell you to stop stuffing your face. The same thing happens if you exercise for extended periods of time; at some point your body will feel exhausted and send the hunger hormone ghrelin to your brain to tell you to gobble more food. The two things expert after expert have told us to do, eat a lot of small meals and exercise more, make us ravenous. Counting calories, taking pictures of our meals, and logging countless hours keeping up food journals is getting us nowhere. We don't have time in our lives to count calories; counting calories is a full-time job that rarely gets any payoff. All along, all we needed to do was exercise moderately, count meals, and know when to eat.

It is said that time exists so everything doesn't happen all at once. I'll agree with that. We place Buffer Zones between our meals so we can allow our bodies to fully ingest and digest our food before we give it another job to do. We must stop asking our bodies to multitask and keep jamming meal after meal into us with no break in between. It's as important to know when to eat as it is to know when not to eat. Last I checked, Americans have two problems, not one. It isn't just that we need to lose weight, but we have to know how to stop gaining any more weight than we already have. Until we stop gaining weight, we will never be able to lose and keep off all the unwanted pounds. The reason so many people end up on yo-yo diets, (gain weight, lose weight, gain weight) is because they never grasped how and why weight gets stored and trapped in the body in the first place and how to stop that from getting out of hand again. That brings us to the next Being Healthy question that will change our lives.

5. How can I stop overproduction of fat?

We already know that Americans are having way too many eating events (meals and snacks). We know this because the average American is carrying around an extra twenty-three pounds of unnecessary fat. It can't be because we are eating too little. But before we dive into why Americans, and quite honestly many parts of the world, are dealing with obesity, let's find out what Americans are consuming.

According to the Dietary Guidelines for Americans from Health.gov, the typical male age nineteen or older consumes 2,640 calories a day; the average for a woman is 1,785 calories. Okay, that's fine. That gives us an idea of where our habits take us.

Now let's compare those real numbers with what the U.S. Department of Agriculture recommends (obviously, these numbers must be lower); for men, the USDA recommends 2,000–2,600 calories for sedentary men, 2,200–2,800 calories for moderately active men, and 2,400–3,000 calories for very active men. Hmm, that doesn't seem far off from the numbers we are putting up each day.

Let's check out the recommendations for women. For sedentary women, the USDA recommends 1,600–2,000 calories, for moderately active women 1,800–2,200 calories, and for very active women 2,000–2,400 calories. Once again, the number of calories that we consume and the number of calories recommended seem almost identical!

So why are we overweight? Aha! Because of the way our bodies store inventory and how, if you don't know the right formula to access it, your body will continue to do what it does year in year out: store more fat and lose more lean muscle mass. Did you know that the typical American loses 5 percent of their lean body mass every decade? And guess what its being replaced with? Fat!

So, here's what's going on. As I mentioned earlier, our bodies work on Last In First Out (LIFO) system. This means your body will always grab the easiest form of energy available. If you just had a ham sandwich, your body will always grab the calories from food you just ate or recently ate before it turns to stored fat.

Our bodies want what's easy. Our bodies will exhaust all quickly available calories from the blood stream before it will even think about checking out what's in the storage room. And if your brain can convince you to eat something (instant gratification) every time it feels like it needs a little bit of energy, that's just fine with your mind-body. Eating when we feel tired is a lot easier than allowing our bodies to do what they are designed to do; use reserves between meals. If we don't allow our bodies to do what's right, they will just run on "Just-In Food" and never burn fossil fuels (reserve fuels) that we made in the past. And if we do what's easy all the time? Well, we get fat. How do we stop the cycle? How do we stop the overproduction of fat? Let me explain.

Dealing with Yummy

There are 168 hours in a week, 10,080 minutes. If we take out 8 hours a day for sleep, that leaves us with 112 hours or 6,720 minutes.

If we then divide those minutes by ten eating events a day (seventy a week), we get ninety-six minutes - so that means we are eating or drinking something with calories approximately every hour and a half. At precisely the peak time, your brain gets a signal from the "hunger" hormone ghrelin. *But here's the thing: it's not really a hunger hormone, it's a volume hormone.* Its job is to tell you when your stomach is starting to get empty or when it is empty. It really isn't telling you, "FEED ME OR WE WILL DIE!" No, it's doing exactly what a fuel gauge does in your car; it's telling you how full your stomach is. Considering a stomach isn't typically empty until five hours after you've eaten a full meal, it makes no sense to eat just because you are feeling a little empty or when you see or smell food. What's fascinating is how much greater our bodies are than our cars. When our car's fuel tank tells us we are on empty, we have to get to a gas station ASAP. But not our bodies.

Our bodies have two fuel tanks; one in our liver and muscles that can deliver all the energy our bodies need at a moment's notice, and the ultimate back-up fuel tank in our adipose tissue that kicks in when fuel tank #1 (liver and muscle storage of glycogen) is partially empty. Our stomach, which we think is a fuel tank, isn't! It's just a *processing center*, along with the small intestine. Its job is to break down our food into the fuel we need.

Let me give you an example: Let's say you just ate 1,100 calories of food. Well, we know it goes into the stomach where it goes through the first press/processing. Fat gets broken down into fatty acids, protein into amino acids, and carbohydrates into glucose. Then the main job of the small intestine is absorption. Practically all the absorbing of nutrients happens here. It can take up to three hours to finish its job.

Now remember, you ate 1,100 calories. Do you think your body needs all those calories at once? Nah, it maybe needs a hundred. So, where do the other calories go? They go to your actual fuel tank: your liver and your muscles. Our stomach is not—I repeat, is not—our fuel tank. The fact that it is partially empty or totally empty has no bearing on how much fuel we have in the tank. That's determined by how much fuel we carry in our liver and muscles. Our liver-and-muscles fuel tank can keep us going for eight to twelve hours, and that's after having just 1,100 calories!

But how often are we eating? Every one and a half hours because our stomachs feel empty. If it bugs you that your stomach feels empty and you want the ghrelin hormone to shut up a little, just drink some water. Remember: your stomach doesn't have a calorie counter, only volume sensors.

Now let's take this example a little further. Let's say you continue not to add any new fuel (food) after eight to twelve hours? Then what? Well, then we can honestly say your real liver-and-muscles fuel tank is close to being empty.

But wait! Our bodies have *two* fuel tanks! The second one is in our adipose tissue that holds triglycerides (concentrated fatty acid tissue) that can take over running the body. One percent of fat fuel can keep your body running for three days! And remember we all tend to have over 30 percent body fat. *Us* starve? Real hunger? Nah. Our bodies were designed to be filled up only occasionally because, back in the day, we didn't know when our next meal was going to be. Having a stomach and small intestine to process and distribute nutrients to our fuel tanks, one for immediate energy needs for the next eight to twelve hours and one for long-term energy needs is genius!

So, why aren't we using our second fuel tank? Why are we eating every one and a half hours when we clearly don't need to? By the way, any food beyond the first one thousand calories we eat in any given meal that isn't needed will be stored as fat. The first one thousand calories go into our primary fuel tank in the liver and muscles, and any calories after that get deposited in the adipose tissue. So what's the reason we eat so much? Simple: food tastes good.

Buffer Zones and Disneyland

So how do we deal with yummy? How do we negotiate with a slice of delicious chocolate cake? Easy, we bargain with it. Think of the five levels of grief: denial, anger, bargaining, depression, and acceptance. The grief we are dealing with is our obsession with food.

Think about how we get fat; when we get an impulse for food, we eat. Do we wait to eat? Only if we have to. And because we are eating willy-nilly, anytime we want, we start getting fat. The first sign is our clothes don't fit; we go into denial, and keep eating. Then the clothes won't go on, we get angry but still keep eating. Then we bargain with ourselves; we will do a little cutting back on our intake of food. It makes little or no difference. We get depressed and resume eating. Then we finally have a choice, either accept being unhealthy (fat) or do something about it. That's where we are now. Food is running our lives. That ends today.

If you are going to be successful in managing your weight, there is only one thing you will need to do, and it isn't to give up the foods you love. It's knowing when it's okay to eat what you want and knowing when to wait to eat what you want. It may sound too good to be true, but that's all Buffer Zones are; time periods when you are not allowed to eat and times you are allowed to eat. If we place the right amount of time between our meals and schedule when we can eat decadently and when we should eat responsibly, we can finally free ourselves from being slaves to food.

Food's only power over us comes from avoidance. Any type of food we avoid because we think it's bad for us we instantly crave. If we want to live in harmony with food, we have to stop calling some of it "guilty pleasures." We should never feel guilty to allow ourselves pleasure. But we can't go overboard. Just because we can have chocolate cake doesn't mean we can have it 24/7.

On July 17, 1955, Disneyland Resort was opened in Anaheim, California. It was the only theme park that was directly designed and built under the supervision of Walt Disney. After the park opened, it began collapsing under its own success. The lines for the rides seemed endless. People and families became agitated by the long waits. When the problem was pointed out to Disney, his staff recommended to keep adding more attractions to meet the demand, but instead of listening to his engineers, Disney went out to talk to the visitors who stood in the long lines to see if the wait was ruining the experience. After a few days of talking to visitor after visitor, the genius Walt Disney discovered that he didn't need to grow the place to keep people happy, because it turned out that what was upsetting everyone wasn't the wait itself but not knowing how long the wait would be. People would be willing to stand in line for hours as long as they knew (1) they were making progress and (2) there was a ride at the end of the wait (a reward). He immediately installed signs to let people know how long the wait was from where they stood in line.

The problem with our eating habits isn't that we are eating the wrong things, it's that we are eating them anytime we want.

We have to be willing to wait to eat some foods, and as Disney showed us, we will be willing to wait, as long as we know how long the wait is. Remember the first law of weight management: satisfaction goes up when caloric intake goes up (big meal) but less frequently (Buffer Zone). As it turns out, all Americans (or really, just about anyone) need is just one really truly delicious meal a day and one or two primer meals to keep us energized. How do we keep from overproducing an inventory of fat? *Eat less meals that mean more to us.* Then allow our bodies during downtime to burn fat as fuel. If we do that, we have mastered food, not the other way around.

6. *How can I deal with over processed food?*

"If it goes bad, it's good for you," the old saying goes. Of course, we are talking about food. If you walk into a grocery store and there isn't an expiration date on the food you're thinking about buying, you can bet it's been processed. It can be canned, bottled, frozen, or have so many preservatives that even the package of Oreo cookies you love may be good for over a year. I used to think any can of Campbell's soup could never go bad (turns out, there is an expiration date on the can). Our ability to add shelf life to food and even alter the identity of food has allowed us to feed over seven billion people on the planet. I'm not saying everyone gets a decent meal, but if we didn't process foods to some degree, we'd never be able to feed our growing population.

For years now, as a society we go through food crazes. At one point, we announced a war on fat and looked to eliminate it from our diet. Food manufacturers started pumping out low-fat foods. Then someone somewhere told us gluten was bad and gluten-free products started showing up. And so it was with high-fructose corn syrup, all-natural, low sodium, zero calorie, etc.

We want quick fixes and we want tasty. If there were a poster child for over processed food, it would be a Twinkie. I've been told that when the end times come there will only be two things that survive: cockroaches and Twinkies. And I'm told that even the cockroach won't go near the Twinkie. Is that how he survived? A serving of Twinkies has 290 calories (23 percent of your daily allowance for saturated fats, 14 percent for total fat), 400 milligrams of sodium (17 percent of daily allowance), and 35 grams of sugar (16 percent of your daily allowance).

Over-processed? That's easy; let's look at the ingredients: enriched bleached wheat flour, flour, reduced iron, B vitamins, niacin, thiamine mononitrate (B1), riboflavin (B2), folic acid, water, sugar, corn syrup, high-fructose corn syrup, partially hydrogenated vegetable and/or animal shortening, soybean, cottonseed and/or canola oil, beef fat, whole eggs, dextrose, etc. There are over forty other ingredients I spared you from having to read. Over-processed? Yep. Will it kill you? No.

Let's look at the other end of the spectrum, something we can all agree is healthy for us. Ever heard of kale? How about broccoli? Or cauliflower? Just about any nutritionist will tell you that these foods are on the "good guy" list. But wait, aren't they over processed, too? Yes, they sure are. The thing these three plants have in common is the humble mustard weed. Man reengineered the life code of that little weed and gave us three brand new products. How wonderful! Better diet through intelligent design! Under-processed or over-processed—heck, even if the apple you eat was sliced for you, that adds one more step to the "process."

I'll repeat what I said before: too much or too little of anything can be bad for you. Did you know you can even die from drinking too much water? Don't worry, unless you're in some insane school fraternity and they are forcing you to drink gallon after gallon of water, you've got nothing to worry about. My point is, eating "all fat" is probably not good for you. But that goes for "all carbs" or "all protein," too. When your stomach gets a balanced amount of each at meals (10 to 35 percent protein—average 15 percent; 45 to 65 percent carbohydrates—average 55 percent; and 30 percent fats) you're good. The key here is to blend. Can some of the food be over-processed? Sure, but as long as they are mixed with a little less processed, you'll be fine.

In a later chapter, we discuss the proper way to not only load your plate, but why the order you eat what you eat may make the biggest difference in you getting your health back. For now, let's focus on the main culprit that's making us all fat and how we can turn our archenemy into our ally! Of course, I'm talking about our desires.

7. How do I make my desire for food work for me instead of against me?

Many years ago, I was watching a comedian on TV who told a funny/sad joke. Let me set it up for you. The man was the size of a tractor trailer, he wore a western shirt that was being stretched to its capacity by a barrel of a chest, and a beer belly so large that if he laid in the surf on the beach and was suddenly surrounded by water from the crest of a wave, his belly would still break the surface of the water and look like a small island. He wore

Levi's blue jeans and you could just barely make out a belt buckle that peeked out from underneath his belly that overlapped it. The man's neck was so large and broad it seemed to just blend away into his shoulders. His cheeks were puffed out like Santa Claus's, red and rosy. He had at least a three-day-old beard. His eyes looked jaundiced.

When he began to talk, you could see his teeth were a mixture of white and yellow like someone had served you a sunny-side-up egg and broken the yolk. In one hand he held a can of beer and had a conversation with it; the audience was merely a fly on the wall allowed to listen.

"You've cost me my car, my TV, my house. You've cost me my job, my money, my savings. You've cost me my wife, my kids, my health. I've lost everything because of you . . ."

There seemed like an incredibly long pregnant pause; it appeared as if he was waiting for a response from the can of beer. When suddenly he smiled, and said, "Oh, what the hell, I'll give you another chance," and drank a large gulp of beer.

That sad and pathetic joke encapsulates in a nutshell our relationship with food. Our love/hate relationship with it. And the reason I believe we have a love/hate relationship with food isn't because food is evil. It isn't. It's what we do with food that's wrong. We eat not because we are hungry, not because we are starving or need nutrition. We eat for so many more reasons than what food is intended for. We eat because we are sad, we eat because we are happy. We eat because we are bored, lonely, or overwhelmed. We eat to feel better, to make some hurt go away, and because for just a quick second, that sugar/fat/salt/sweet/sour high feels so good, so we keep eating. We are medicating ourselves with food. And it's killing us. We are eating our emotions instead of dealing with them. We are hiding from instead of confronting our problems. And when we hide out into the bunkers of our life, we take munchies.

Emotions are driving us to overeat and its only emotions that will free us from our nightmare. Logic won't save us. We have to fight fire with fire.

Emotional Hunger versus Physical Hunger

Fortunately for us, there are well-documented warning signs that present themselves before we go on an emotional eating binge. If we look out for these signs before gobbling up that chocolate iced donut that just popped into your mind because it was left over from yesterday's caravan to Krispy Kreme, we can stop the cycle of emotional eating. If we don't look out for the warning signs, our brains typically reason with us like this: "It would be a shame for it to go to waste. Seriously, it's going to be eaten eventually anyway, why not just put that little guy out of its misery now?"

Of course, the reason we can't let those thoughts drive us is because if we go to the kitchen and eat that lone donut, it's unlikely there will be any healthy food eaten with it. I doubt you'll say, "Hmm, I'll have a piece of broccoli with my donut to balance the scales." No, you won't. You'll just eat that donut, and as a result, without food blending, your insulin level will spike and then drop within thirty minutes—then have a food craving all over again.

Don't forget, when you eat is as important as what you eat. If when that donut craving popped into your head you said, "Wait, it's just x number of hours until my next meal, and I can have that donut as my dessert after I've loaded my stomach correctly [I'll explain what "food loading" is soon] and then I can have my donut minus the insulin spike," you've done good. No diet will be successful if you are denied food forever. The Buffer Zone just teaches you to delay the gratification so your body can be healthy.

So, what are the warning signs that tell you that you are emotionally eating and letting environmental triggers drive you to eat when your body already has full gas tanks?

Emotional Eating Red Flags

1. *It's been less than three hours since you've had a meal.* You're not hungry! Even if your stomach is growling it just means your stomach is telling you its capacity status. Don't forget your stomach is a processing center and your small intestine is a distribution center. Your actual gas tank in your liver and muscles holds eight to twelve hours of fuel or approximately one thousand calories for any type of emergency. If your first tank is empty, your body can run on fat fuel. One percent of fat fuel lasts three days. You aren't starving.

2. *Real hunger builds slowly, not suddenly.* If you just suddenly feel like you are starving, you are in the grips of emotional hunger. The need for instant gratification = emotional hunger.

3. *Emotional hunger is a picky eater.* If you are only hungry for a specific food, the emotional monster has you by the throat—or rather, stomach. True hunger will be in the mood to eat almost anything.

4. *Emotional hunger is driven by thoughts in your head and not by any physical demands.* If the craving is coming from your mind rather than from your body, the craving is driven by a stressor you'd rather avoid. And what better way to do that than with a tub of ice cream? Don't give in! Delay!

5. *Once you start eating, you can't stop until it hurts.* Mindful eating that keeps checking in to see when you are satisfied gets sidelined by the thought, "MUST EAT MORE!" Emotional eating has no control.

6. *When you've finished eating and you collect all the empty plates, emotional eating feels shame.* True hunger that has just been satisfied feels content. If shame is following your meals, emotion is driving your appetite and your life.

Psychoanalyst Nina Savelle-Rocklin says, "Food is not the true problem. Food is actually a solution to the problem, albeit a damaging one. If your boss turns you down for a promotion and you eat ice cream for comfort, then the real problem is your disappointment and resentment. Ice cream is a way of temporarily coping. Overeating can also express emotional states. If you are lonely, food symbolically fills a void. If you are mad at yourself for what you just ate, maybe you displaced your anger toward others onto yourself. The good news is that when you address the underlying reasons for 'why' you are eating, instead of focusing on 'what' you are eating, those food issues disappear."

So, how do we break free? How do we stop all the stress eating? Simple: by using the same desires that are driving us to eat to drive us to be healthy. We make desire chains.

Desire Chains

In 2006 William B. Irvine wrote the definitive book about desire entitled, *On Desire: Why We Want What We Want*. Here's a quote from François de La Rochefoucauld that appears in his book:

> *"Man often thinks he is in control when he is being controlled, and while his mind is striving in one direction his heart is imperceptibly drawing him in another."*

Mr. Irvine candidly points out in his book that we aren't as complicated as we may think we are. Our desires are all rooted in one principle: "Do what feels good and avoid feeling bad." You will recall we touched on the pleasure principle earlier. But the problem with this seemingly straightforward principle is this: What if what feels good now will make me feel bad later? "A second on the lips forever on the hips." Couldn't say that any plainer. What we do now always has consequences. Obviously, it's more fun to spend every dollar we make, but when it comes time to retire, we don't have the savings to do so. Only one out of twenty Americans will have enough money to retire in the lifestyle they have been accustomed to when they get to their golden years. Tasty can end up bitter. So, what are we to do?

Well, according to Mr. Irvine, we have to construct desire chains. What's a desire chain? It's any emotionally anchored group of action steps that leads to the reward we desire. For example: A young child goes to his mom and dad and says he wants the latest video game, so he asks for sixty dollars. If the parent simply gave the child the money, that would create a short desire chain. Count the steps.

1. Desire for new video game created after seeing the commercial advertised on TV. Child imagines how much fun he will have while playing the game. Brain gives itself marching orders: "Get that video game!"

2. Child checks personal finances (money in pocket) and finds a dollar and a quarter. Child feels sad. Brain doesn't like feeling sad and still wants fun and looks for the shortest distance to get desire satisfied—(i.e., ask parents for the money)!

3. Child asks parents for money. Parents give child money and child feels excited, imagining himself playing the game already.

4. New problem: child needs ride to the store to buy the video game. No transportation! Child feels sad again and returns to his parents for help.

5. Child asks parents to take him to the store, and his parents agree.

6. Parents take the child to the store and luckily the game is in stock and is purchased.

7. Child returns home and plays the game.

Believe it or not, this is a short desire chain. Mind you, at any point it could have become longer. For starters, the parents could have refused to pay for the new video game and the child might have had to save up the money. Or perhaps the parents may not have been able to drive the child to the store right away and child would have to wait until the weekend. Or even worse, the child might have had to earn the money and find his own transportation to the store, only to find the video game sold out.

Things we absolutely desire are called "terminal desires." These are things we are willing to go through hell and high water for. The action steps required to achieve the terminal desire (in this case, the video game) are called "instrumental desires," because those action steps are instrumental in getting what is desired.

If we eat every time our brain creates a desire, will we be healthy? No. What if we just tell our brains "No! No bad food for you! No more bread, no more pasta, no more sweets. They are bad! No more." No, that won't work. Willpower is a limited resource. Eventually you will run out and eat what you are avoiding. But willpower is strong enough to deal with a delay. In fact, we are designed and built to deal with delays. Heck, we all deal with delays every day! From traffic, to standing in lines or waiting for a meeting to start. We are prepared to deal with delays as long as we are granted our terminal desire (i.e., our video game).

Like I said before, no food (and that includes a Twinkie) is so bad that it can't be eaten, just as long as its blended with healthier food. So the trick to being healthy is very straightforward; add one action step between what you desire and the instrumental desires it takes to acquire it. All we have to do is add a Buffer Zone. Every day on the Buffer Zone Diet you will get a meal of your choosing, so all I ask is when that food craving pops into your head you tell yourself that you just have to wait until the next big meal to have it. Which means you are always within twenty-four hours of getting what you want! And if that's all you have to do is learn to patiently wait to get the food you desire and do ten minutes of strength training and thirty minutes of cardio a day, isn't it worth it to be healthy? I would think so.

In the next chapter, I'm going to lay out the entire plan and formula at the heart of the Buffer Zone. The formula is over 116 years old and we can thank the father of quantum mechanics, Max Planck, for showing us the light!

CHAPTER 8

The Equation

Realizing the human body was an assembly line led me to the Three Environmental Pillars *(Muda, Muri, Mura)* that clearly indicate environment regulates behavior. If your environment is in chaos you won't be able to take care of yourself. Order your environment and remove any unnecessary waste before you take on your body.

Once you're out of panic mode you can embrace *The Four Laws of Weight Management*:

I.   **SATISFACTION INCREASES:** Calories go up per meal and frequency of meals goes down.

II. **SATISFACTION DECREASES:** Calories go down per meal and frequency of meals goes up.

III. **BODY FAT INCREASES:** Calories go down per meal and frequency of meals goes up.

IV. **BODY FAT DECREASES:** Calories go up per meal and frequency of meals goes down.

Then by asking the right questions (the ones we asked in Chapter 7), we can deduce *The Seven Truths of Creation* that support The Four Laws.

They are:

1. When you deliver food to your body is as important as what you deliver. (Time)

2. Only fill up your gas tank when it's empty. (Space)

3. "Nothing happens until something moves." — Einstein (Momentum)

4. The time between the meals is as important as the meals themselves. (Nothing)

5. The best way to access reserves is to cut production. (Scarcity)

6. Use sequencing and food blending to allow your processing center (stomach) to create healthy fuel (chyme) that is optimal for running your body. (Fusion)

7. Don't fight your desire for food. Use your desires to help you have fewer meals that mean more to you. (Choice)

But even after all my progress, I believed there had to be one unifying formula, one theory of everything, that tied it all together. In cosmology, the theory of everything has been the long-sought-out holy grail since Einstein told us of the special law of relativity. One theory to unify the four forces; strong force, weak force, electromagnetic, and gravity. An elegant equation that could bring the world of the small and the world of the large together.

While that equation has never been found, I believe there also has to be one elegant equation that regulates the weight of the human body. I'd discovered The Three Environmental Pillars, The Four Laws of Weight Management, and The Seven Truths of Creation that we could implement into our lives to design our perfect diet for a lifetime. I had all the pieces in front of me, now all I had to do was tie it all together. What was the Unified Theory of Weight? I had to find it.

Weighty Matters

In science and engineering it is understood that the weight of an object is the force on that object due to gravity. To put it technically, the weight of an object is equal to the product of the mass (m) and the magnitude of the local gravitational acceleration (g). $W = mg$. There is very little we can do about the force of gravity as long as we live on Earth, so there is no adjusting our weight by tinkering with that part of the equation. That just leaves us with mass. If we want to adjust our weight, we have to change our mass. But what is our mass? What is mass? Here's what Wikipedia has to say:

"In physics, mass is a property of a physical body. It is generally a measure of an object's resistance to changing its state of motion when a force is applied. It is determined by the strength of its mutual gravitational attraction to other bodies, its resistance to acceleration or directional changes, and in the theory of relativity gives the mass-energy content of a system. In Newtonian physics, mass can be generalized as the amount of matter in an object."

Whether that all sounds like a lot of mumbo jumbo or not (I'm not a physicist; even I had to read it over a few times) is irrelevant. What I'd like you to focus on is the last sentence from the quote: "Mass can be generalized as the amount of matter in an object." That's the money sentence! If eating too much adds more "matter" to our bodies and not eating at all reduces the matter from our bodies, then what is the perfect equation that would allow us to control our matter so we could control our weight? Put even simpler, what was the right interval that a body needed to have more matter added to it (fed) that would allow the owner of that body to be happy with it? It clearly wasn't three to six meals a day! If that was the case, we would all be trim. No, the *frequency* at which a body should be fed had to be at the core of the equation I was looking for.

In 2012, Ian Stewart (a man far more brilliant than me) wrote a marvelous book (for normal people like us) titled *In Pursuit of the Unknown: 17 Equations That Changed the World*. It's where I turned when I went looking for my equation for weight/mass realignment. With each turn of the page, Mr. Stewart takes us on incredible journeys through the unknown. We learn about Pythagoras's Theorem, calculus, Newton's law of gravity, wave equations, Maxwell's equations, and thermodynamics. The book is plain English to nonscientific folk. But where the book raised my spidey senses was in chapter 14: "Quantum Weirdness, Schrodinger's Equation." The equation doesn't just see matter as a particle, but as a wave and explains how matter waves can be distributed.

Knowing how a body reacts to matter, how matter had this dual personality (particle/wave duality) had me scratching my head. "Let's see: matter is like one hundred thousand fans at a football stadium, each standing at the exact time required to produce a beautiful-looking wave all around the stadium up until the wave function collapses and everybody goes back to acting individually." Why did it "matter" to me that photons that I couldn't see and measure would have any effect on the management of weight loss and a healthy body? Was I trying to make a square peg fit into a round hole? Quantum mechanics should have nothing to do with the mass of a human body but something was telling me otherwise. I knew the frequency of meals was central to balancing our weight and I knew that a meal was nothing more than a packet of calories that was delivered to the body.

And there! That's when I saw it, probably the way Einstein saw it in 1905 when he explained the photoelectric effect. A "quanta" or quantity of electricity could determine how much energy a bundle had. These bundles or packets of energy contained photons. What if I replaced photons in the equations for calories? What if counting calories was wrong and all we should be counting is the magnitude of meals (packets of calories). Maybe calories in and calories out wasn't the key to weight management, maybe all we had to know was how and when those packets of calories were being propagated into the system. Was it possible that how the calories are received by the body could affect the rate of consumption and weight retention? How could it be possible that what we thought about what we ate could have any effect on what we ate or how it would be processed? Particle/wave duality told me that all possibilities are in play when it comes to the quantum world. Could the same be said of food? The answer is yes.

Lighten Up

In 1894, an electrical company hired a German physicist named Max Planck to design the most efficient light bulb possible, a light bulb that would produce the most light and consume the least amount of energy. The key to solving this puzzle was one of radiation. In physics, *radiation* is defined as the emission of energy in the form of waves/particles through a medium.

Translation: If we run electricity through a light bulb, it should radiate light. The question then is, how is the intensity of the light bulb dependent on the frequency of the radiation and its temperature? And when the temperature of that bulb stayed on bright for a long enough period of time, it burnt itself out. Handling energy was no laughing matter. What Max Planck quickly figured out was how energy depended on frequency. And frequency wasn't just one big whole thing. It wasn't a continuum. It was made up of multiples of the frequency separated by little tiny gaps.

Think of a dotted line versus a straight line. And these little dotted lines had to be constant, they had to have the same energy.

While this constant was originally called the proportionality constant, we now refer to it as Planck's Constant (denoted by the letter h). It literally measures the minimal increment of energy at $6.62607004 \times 10^{-34}$ in joules.

Okay, I know I'm losing you (except you brainiacs). What Planck had figured out was that energy was equal to the product of that minimal energy increment and its frequency. So, I'll strip the fancy jargon with words anyone can relate to. *Your mass, your weight, is regulated by the number of minimal or maximum energy increments (meals) multiplied by the frequency of those meals.*

> *Example:* A lot of maximum energy (high-calorie) meals given in a set time period makes mass go up. That, I am sure you know. But what I bet you didn't know is this: a lot of minimum energy (low-calorie) meals given in a set time also makes mass go up! You see? It's not the size of the meal that is the trigger to weight gain, it's the frequency! WE ARE JUST EATING WAY TOO FREQUENTLY.

The equation that Max Planck came up with is $E = h\nu$; energy equals Planck's constant times frequency. That was the equation I was looking for! E represented the mass we wanted to control. h represented the caloric intake of each meal we would consume and ν (pronounced *nu*, from the Greek alphabet) represented the frequency we needed to follow in order to control our weight. *How often and when we eat was the holy grail that would allow us to break free from our dependency on food!* Now, all I had to do was experiment with the equation to figure out what were the frequency numbers I needed a day/week and how to bundle the caloric load of each meal to optimize the health of the human body. It would soon be guinea-pig time and there would need to be some preparation before I began experiments on myself.

Be Prepared!

If I expected to have any success with The Buffer Zone Diet I figured I'd better review what I knew, thought I knew, and didn't know. So, I compiled three lists. I started with what I was certain of in terms of weight management.

List 1: What I Know

1. A lot of small meals each day doesn't help lose weight in the long term.

2. Trying to eat just a "snack" doesn't solve my food cravings. Eating anything just makes me hungrier than before I ate. Eating increases my appetite unless satiety (feeling full) is achieved. **Snacks serve no purpose.**

3. It's difficult to manage a bunch of small meals a day without it interfering with my work flow. Lots of meals gobbles up/wastes my time.

4. If after I eat a meal I don't feel satisfied, I will get food cravings shortly after my meal (within thirty minutes).

5. Even after I have a satisfying meal I will get a new food thought at approximately one hour after the meal. The new craving will pop into my head strongly for the next thirty minutes, then diminish to a faint signal for the next hour and a half (three hours total). Then, depending on the size of the meal, I will get scattered food thoughts for the next two hours (five hours total). After my stomach is empty (after five hours) the food craving thoughts have little effect on me. It's as if my fake food cravings had given up.

6. If I haven't eaten anything for eight hours (the beginning of when my fuel tank in my liver and muscles is starting to run low) I actually get my first no-kidding hunger pangs. Between the eighth and tenth hour, our bodies are transitioning to use fat fuel, triglycerides.

7. If I wake up in the morning and it's been over ten hours since my last meal (body is on fat fuel) I don't wake up hungry.

8. If I skip a breakfast because I'm not hungry, I tend to be hungrier at lunch.

9. If I eat a small, well-designed meal at lunch, even if I've skipped breakfast, I feel satisfied.

10. If I eat three small meals in a row over the course of the day, by the third meal I no longer

feel satisfied. *Conclusion:* the maximum number of small meals in a row that I can have to stay satisfied is two. After that, my body craves for a full-tank meal (over one thousand calories) or I won't feel satisfied.

11. The speed at which I eat affects how much I eat.

12. The order in which I eat the food affects how much I eat.

13. My body weight fluctuates greatly throughout the day (three- to four-pound swings).

14. Working out was less important than I originally believed. The amount of exercise I need to be healthy turned out to be ten minutes a day of strength training and thirty minutes of cardio.

15. If I didn't put enough time between my last meal of today and my first meal of the day tomorrow, I'd never burn away fat fuel.

16. If I don't get enough sleep, I get more food cravings during the subsequent day.

17. I think better on an empty stomach.

18. If I don't stay hydrated I get dizzy and constipated.

19. I have to drink water throughout the day instead of trying to drink a lot in one sitting or I wouldn't stay hydrated.

20. Diet soda made me thirstier and hungrier.

List 2: What I Thought I Knew

1. I believed that the success of weight management was going to be 80 percent "less meals that mean more to you" and 20 percent exercise.

2. I believed that rapid weight loss was not only unhealthy but not a long-term plan.

3. I believed a goal of one pound a week weight loss was a sensible goal.

4. I believed it was important to have a digital scale that would be more accurate than an analog scale.

5. I believed that since my weight fluctuated so much on a daily basis, there had to be a better system to measure my weight than just what the scale told me.

6. I believed I needed to vary my workout or my body would adapt and the exercise wouldn't have long-term effects.

7. I believed that there couldn't just be one Buffer Zone Diet that everyone followed.

8. I believed there had to be ways to adjust the Buffer Zone to combat plateaus that arrive in any diet.

9. I believed that we had trained ourselves to feel hungry when our stomachs were empty (which isn't true) and that we could rewire our brains

to feel happy and content with empty stomachs but with full fuel tanks (glycogen stores in liver and muscles and fat fuel).

10. I believed that the average person should run their bodies on 60 to 80 percent glycogen stores (just in calories or just in food or new food) and on 20 to 40 percent triglycerides (fat fuel) on a weekly basis.

11. I believed that if I blended food correctly that I could stop labeling any food as bad food.

12. I believed that the best way to start any full-tank meal is with a salad and glass of water.

13. I believed that one should make every attempt in the world to not skip breakfast, but if it happened occasionally, we would survive.

14. I believed lunch was the most important meal of the day, not breakfast.

15. I believed that lunch should under no circumstances be skipped.

16. I believed late afternoon naps interfered with my nighttime sleep.

17. I believed green drinks were a waste of money.

18. I believed I gained more fat when I overindulged protein versus carbs.

19. I believed that food was the primary way people sedated themselves for comfort.

20. I believed picky eaters were risk averse and I believed there were hidden dangers to being risk averse.

21. I believed if you didn't love the diet you are on, Buffer Zone or otherwise, you would never stick with it. The diet had to fit your lifestyle, not the other way around.

List 3: What I Didn't Know

1. I didn't know the facts of nutrition. Plan: take a thirty-six-lecture course on nutrition from the Teaching Company. Title of course: *Nutrition Made Clear* taught by Professor Roberta H. Anding, Baylor College of Medicine and Texas Children's Hospital. She has a master of science in nutrition and is a registered dietician, a certified diabetes educator, and is a certified specialist in sports dietetics. She is the director of sports nutrition in the Adolescent Medicine and Sports Medicine Clinic at the Baylor College of Medicine and Texas Children's Hospital Department of Pediatrics, and she teaches in the Department of Kinesiology at Rice University. She also serves as the dietician for the Houston Texans.

2. I didn't know the facts of the human body. Plan: Take a thirty-two-lecture course on the human

body from the Teaching Company. Title of the course: *Understanding the Human Body: An Introduction to Anatomy and Physiology* taught by Professor Anthony Goodman, MD, FACS, Montana State University. He is an adjunct professor in the Department of Microbiology at Montana State University. Previously, he was clinical associate professor of surgery at the University of Miami School of Medicine. He received his bachelor of arts from Harvard College and his medical doctorate from Cornell Medical College. He is a fellow of the American College of Surgeons and a Diplomate of the American Board of Surgery.

3. I didn't know the eating habits of Americans.

4. I didn't know all the reasons why people choose the food they eat.

5. I didn't know what organizations I could trust to tell me unbiased information on nutrition.

6. I hadn't read all the top diet books to see what experts agreed were the facts about nutrition and what were nothing more than fad diets. Plan: read top twenty best-selling books on diets looking for universal facts.

7. I didn't know the body mass index off the top of my head.

8. I didn't know what metabolic syndrome is.

9. I didn't know about the digestive tract.

10. I didn't know about probiotics.

11. I didn't know how stress could alter the nervous system.

12. I didn't completely understand all the factors that could affect one's basal metabolic rate.

13. I didn't know about the thermic effect of food.

14. I didn't know which equation was the best to determine an individual's ideal body weight given that individual's sex and height.

15. I didn't know about Non-Exercise Activity Thermogenesis (NEAT).

16. I didn't know all the functions of water.

17. I didn't know how to correctly test my hydration level.

18. I didn't know the signs of being dehydrated.

19. I didn't know how long it took my body to acclimate to a new body weight low.

20. I didn't know everything about carbohydrates.

21. I didn't know everything about protein.

22. I didn't know everything about fats.

23. I didn't know about the glycemic index.

24. I didn't know everything about fiber.

25. I didn't know how much fiber I needed.

26. I didn't know what my daily protein, carb, and fat requirements were.

27. I didn't know the dangers of saturated fats and trans fats.

28. I didn't know what trans fats were.

29. I didn't know the benefits of unsaturated fats.

30. I didn't know about vitamins and minerals.

31. I didn't know the connection between an improper diet and cardiovascular disease.

32. I didn't truly understand obesity.

33. I didn't know about Type 1 or Type 2 diabetes.

34. I didn't know all the connections between diet and cancer.

35. I didn't know how to read a food label.

36. I didn't know the health benefits of organic food.

37. I didn't know how supplements could affect the human body.

38. I didn't have a hard fact list that anybody could use to understand how to nourish the human body.

39. I didn't know the cardiovascular system.

40. I didn't know the respiratory system.

41. I didn't know the nervous system.

42. I didn't know the reproductive system.

43. I didn't know the musculoskeletal system.

44. I didn't know the immune system.

45. In general, I didn't know why people got cancer.

46. I didn't know the endocrine system.

47. I didn't know the urinary system.

48. And finally, I had to accept I didn't know what I didn't know. There were bound to be things along my journey that I would learn about subjects I didn't even know existed. I had to accept and be open to all new data that came my way. I had my Three Environmental Pillars, the Four Laws of Weight Management, the Seven Truths of Creation, Planck's Equation, and I have my three action lists. It was time to roll up my sleeves, start my diet, answer the questions that I didn't know, and prove or disprove the things I thought I knew. I only had this one life and I had to start living it, and that required a healthy body. Let the games begin!

CHAPTER 9

Guinea Pig, Part 1

According to the Hamwi Equation, I should weigh 178 pounds (male, six feet tall. 106 pounds for the first five feet and six pounds for each additional inch). I was 216 pounds. I had thirty-eight pounds to lose. It was Saturday, October 31, 2015; my start date was the very next day, November 1. If I could stick to my goal of one pound a week, I would be on a journey of nine and a half months—until a little after Independence Day 2016. I should have my own independence from food.

Once I knew what weight was healthiest for me, I multiplied my goal weight times ten to establish my baseline minimum calorie intake to satisfy my basal metabolic rate (minimum number of calories to operate my body even if I laid perfectly still in bed with my eyes open).

178 × 10 = 1,780

I needed 1,780 calories to just stay alive. I couldn't go under that or I might hurt myself. Then, since I wasn't sure how active I was, I placed myself in the sedentary camp and multiplied 1,780 calories by 1.3, which equals 2,314 calories. I had been and still do work out every day but I also sit at a desk all day. Then I multiplied 2,314 calories × 7 days in the week to get 16,198 calories per week. This was my max. If I wanted to reach my goal, I would have to stay under this number, week in and week out.

Next I needed a schedule. I knew too many meals was America's problem, but how many was I going to have?

To answer this, I spent a few weeks prior calculating precisely how many calories were in the meals that I loved: wife's lasagna, her New York-style hot dogs, shepherd's pie, etc. And I calculated that they varied anywhere from 1,300 to 1,500 calories easy and with extra helpings over 2,000. I'd have to watch my extra helpings.

So, I divided 16,198 by 1,500 calories and I got 10.8 full-tank meals (over one-thousand-calorie meals). *Hmm*, I thought, *that's not enough meals for a week*. But then I realized that after I had a full-tank meal, my next two meals didn't have to be as big to satisfy me. They were more like bridge meals to help get me along, a hop and skip to jump to my big meal. Then that settled it: I'd use 7 out of 10.8 big meals so I could have 1 a day. That left me with 3.8 meals at 1,500 calories each, which equaled 5,700 calories. I divided 5,700 by the 7 days in the week and got 814 calories extra per day for my bridge meals (that I would later call primer meals because their job was to keep me in my prime so that I could keep my power up). Of the allotted 814 calories extra a day, I used 300 for breakfast, 300 for lunch, and I used the remaining 214 calories for the 8 ounces of chocolate milk I drank immediately after my workout. There is quite a bit of literature on the benefits of chocolate milk after a workout for restoring glycogen stores in the muscles.

I labeled my first Buffer Zone plan the 7/14 plan, representing seven main meals a week and fourteen primer meals a week. Okay. I worked out the calories, now I had to work out the timing.

The Buffer Zone is all about *the space between the meal.* If I didn't put enough time between my last meal of the day today and my first meal of the day tomorrow, I'd never make a dent in my body fat. Remember, it takes ten hours of no eating before your body primarily switches to body fat to run your body. My initial belief was our bodies should run on no more than 80 percent of just-in food (jiffy food) and no less than 20 percent fossil fuel (fat fuel). Or to be more specific, 80 percent glycogen fuel, 20 percent triglyceride fuel. If I was going to pull that off I needed to make sure that 20 percent of the 168 hours of the week (33.6 hours or 33 hours and 36 minutes) I was running on fat fuel. This was my plan: I got off work at 5:00 p.m., if after I got home and had my dinner and dessert, I would finish by 6:00 p.m. and then not eat breakfast until 8:48 a.m. That would give me my 4.8 hours of fat-fueling hours per night (I get to 4.8 hours by subtracting the 10 hours it takes for me to get into primary fat fuel mode from a Buffer Zone between 6:00 at night until 8:48 the next morning). A Buffer Zone is any time you are not eating. I had designed a 14.8-hour buffer to get 4.8 hours (or 4 hours and 48 minutes) of benefit.

So that was it; the first ever Buffer Zone plan was in place. I'd eat seven meals a week and fourteen primers. I'd spend 80 percent of my hours on just-in fuel and 20 percent of my hours on fat fuel.

But I still had a few questions: What was I going to eat? When was I going to work out? How was I going to record my progress? When was I going to weigh myself?

Filling in the Blanks

MEALS:

While I know now that 55 percent of my calories should be carbohydrates, 15 to 20 percent of my calories should be protein, and 25 to 30 percent of my calories should be fats (no more than 7 to 10 percent of my calories saturated fats), I didn't know it when I started experimenting with the Buffer Zone. So, when I first designed my meals I tried to keep it as simple as possible.

For my primers (approx. three hundred calories or so), I just planned on having an even portion of my nutrients. For breakfast, I had Trader Joe's steel-cut oatmeal. There are three types of oatmeal out there: whole, rolled, and flakes (instant). Steel-cut oats are the healthiest for you. Whole grains lower your risk of high blood pressure and Type II Diabetes. They also lower your cholesterol (your LDL: Low Density Lipoprotein) that can lead to cardiovascular disease.

The tough part of steel-cut oatmeal is the long preparation time, but Trader Joe's has solved that problem. A copacker does all the hard work for you by making it and freezing it into little hockey pucks. All you have to do is take it out of its vacuum-sealed bag and pop it into the microwave for three minutes. From one hockey puck of steel-cut oatmeal I get 150 calories, 20 from fat, no cholesterol, 4 grams of dietary fiber, 5 grams of protein, and 27 grams of carbohydrates (9 percent of my daily requirement).

Oatmeal is listed by the Mayo Clinic as one of the top five foods for your health. I added to my oatmeal one egg (over easy, and yes I ate the cholesterol-ridden yolk). That was 80 calories. Then I topped it off with a small fruit cup (apples, oranges, grapes, raspberries, melon, and pineapple) a half cup comes in around 70 calories. 150 + 80 + 70 = 300! Perfect! I had designed my primer breakfast. Next my primer lunch.

Once again, I wanted to keep it as easy as possible, so I opted for an open-face sandwich. One slice of bread; whole grain is best for you but if you don't like it try mixed grain. That came in at 85 calories. Then I put a couple of thin slices of turkey (80 calories) and a slice of Colby jack cheese (110 calories) and half an apple (my wife chose Fuji—60 calories). The total came in at 335 calories—a little over, but I didn't sweat it. I also had at least 12 ounces of water with each primer meal. I tried to always drink the water as cold as possible to help burn a few extra calories a day. Interesting note: If you drink 64 ounces of ice cold water a day, you will lose 6.4 pounds by the end of the year! Crazy, huh?! Your body has to expend energy in order to warm up that water. I picked up this tip from a spectacular book called *Mindless Eating* by Brian Wansink, PhD. Brilliant book. I highly recommend it!

My plan was to eat the same primer meals Monday through Friday for breakfast and lunch. Since the job of the primer meal was only to keep essential nutrients in my bloodstream for three to five hours at a time, I didn't want to overthink them. For dinner, I decided I should be allowed to eat what I want (within reason). My fear was second and third helpings that I loved to have. So my plan of attack was to limit the space in my workstation (stomach). If my stomach was full, I wouldn't want second helpings. So, that's when I came up with the idea of "frontloading." I would eat a large salad (mixed greens, some fruits, vegetables, and nuts) with a light vinaigrette and drink a large glass of water (12 ounces) before I ate my main meal. By frontloading with my salad and water it made it easier to be satisfied with one healthy-sized portion of whatever my wonderful wife was cooking and (most importantly) allow me to have dessert! I have a sweet tooth. I always love to end my meal with something yummy. I love caramel nut clusters dipped in chocolate.

For the weekends, I switched things up. My wife and I liked to have our main meal for lunch so dinners on the weekend became primers. Seven delicious meals a week (less meals that mean more to me) and fourteen primers: the 7/14 plan. My meals were set.

Working Out

For as long as I can remember I've had a love-hate relationship with working out. For me, working out wasn't so much something that brought me joy, it was the thing I had to do in order to eat what I wanted and stay "healthy." I can't count the number of injuries I've had while working out. Being a goal-oriented person, I felt obligated to always top my previous workout. This would eventually lead to me breaking. It was a vicious cycle. Prior to the Buffer Zone, I was doing one to one and a half hours of cardio each day and thirty minutes of strength training. I'd have to get up a little after five in the morning to get it all in. I always felt exhausted. And when I felt exhausted, I gravitated toward food for a quick pick-me-up.

One day, about eight months before my "aha" moment about the Buffer Zone, I had my "aha" moment about working out.

"What if more exercise *isn't* good for you? What if less time and more intensity/frequency could be just as good as my two-hour 'pace myself' workouts?"

I had to try. I didn't want to go to a gym and I have adequate workout space in my home, so I looked for an app that could generate short, concise, powerful workouts for me. The app needed to vary the workouts so I wouldn't get bored. After experimenting with different ones for a week, I settled on Fitstar. It costs about ten dollars a month and offers four main workout packages.

1. **Daily Dose:** Quick conditioning, 6-session weekly goal, 10–15 minute sessions. Daily Dose features short sessions to complement a busy lifestyle.

2. **Get Lean:** Trim and tone. 4-session weekly goal, 30–45 minute sessions. Full of fat burning moves, Get Lean is perfect for people who want to lose weight.

3. **Get Moving:** Beginner basics. 2-session weekly goal. 10–20 minute sessions. Get moving is great

for those getting started, offering manageable sessions for anyone.

4. **Get Strong:** Maximize your muscles. 3-session weekly goal. 20–40 minute sessions. Get strong is a blend of body weight and cardio moves ideal for building strength.

I chose Daily Dose. I figured I'd rather work out every day for short periods than three or four days for long periods. When it came to working out, I went in the opposite direction I was going with food. With food, I was having higher volume (caloric) meals but less frequently (one big meal a day). With working out, I was willing to work out more frequently (once a day versus three to four times a week) at a higher intensity, so I wouldn't have to waste time in the gym. I began to realize that for the Buffer Zone to work I had to spend less time eating and less time working out; but when I did, I had to make the most of it.

I realize that everyone has a different schedule for when they want to work out, but for me I like to get it over with. I have always worked out immediately after waking up. I don't like having that workout hanging over my head all day. I picked the same time I would wake up each day—6:50 a.m.—and I'd be good to go. Since I'm a little groggy when I initially wake up, I give myself thirty minutes to get into my home gym. That gives me time to get out of bed, do my daily ritual, and get dressed. By 7:20 a.m. every day I went through my Fitstar workout, which typically took about ten minutes. Then I'd jump onto the treadmill for thirty minutes of cardio. I don't like to run so I walk at a pace of four miles per hour. To walk at a lower speed typically doesn't give you a tough enough cardio workout. I increased the incline, adding hills to make it tougher.

When I was done, it was around eight o'clock, and then I'd weigh myself. This was going to be my new workout routine. Shorter workouts with higher intensity that mean more to me and waste less of my time. Time, if you haven't figured out, is everything.

Weigh-In

If my calculations were correct, the Buffer Zone should target fat, not water or lean muscle mass. It's easy to lose weight if you use diuretics or allow yourself to cannibalize your muscle mass. Since we are mostly made of water, it's easy to design a diet that will force you to lose water weight. Quick weight-loss plans aren't designed for you to be healthy, but to see a sexy number on the scale so you feel good. Once those diets deplete the water from your muscles and glycogen stores, they quickly lose steam. A healthy diet has to allow you to use your just-in food (daily food intake) and stored fuel (fat fuel).

Some of the healthy diets I studied, like the Mediterranean Diet, were great about stopping weight gain but had no real plan to target old fat. It isn't enough to figure out how to stop gaining new body fat if you haven't figured out how to lose old body fat; you'd just be going around in circles. One of my concerns about the Buffer Zone was accuracy of daily measuring. I knew the only way to know if the Buffer Zone was working was to see a weight change on the scale or inches lost on my body (which would be accompanied by looser-fitting clothes). My estimate predicted I'd lose 2 ounces of body fat a day. That's about half a stick of butter or 437.5 calories of body fat (48.6 grams of fat). Even switching to a digital scale wouldn't pick up those slight improvements. Add to the fact that our bodies fluctuate a few pounds a day; it may take me a few weeks to see real weight loss.

I'd heard differing opinions on how often a person should weigh themselves, some "experts" said only once a week, while others said daily. The first thing I had to figure out (loving statistics) was the probability on any given day that the weight on the scale was correct. Of course, I'd weigh myself at the same time, no clothes, on the same scale, every day. But my question was, how many days of weighing in (data) do I need to calculate my true weight? I knew that if I added up my weight for five days and divided it by the number of weigh-ins (five), I could calculate my five-day moving average. I believed my five-day moving average would be closer to my true weight. By averaging my data, I could eliminate the random highs and lows that show up in daily fluctuations due to water retention, poor sleep, too much sodium, or any of the dozen-plus reasons our bodies hold on to weight.

Every time we are stressed, our bodies release cortisol (a stress hormone), which wreaks havoc on our digestive system and water retention. Add to that hormonal cycles, illnesses, injuries, and travel; I calculated that the odds of your weight being your "true weight" on any given day you step on the scale is about one in ten! Then when you calculate that the Buffer Zone would target and remove two ounces of body fat a day, it would take approximately eight days to see one pound come off! I worried that the typical person might quit within two to three weeks after their scales didn't show them any major improvement. The Buffer Zone would remove three to four pounds a month (if you had a lot of weight to lose, twenty or more pounds) and one to two pounds a month (if you needed to lose less than ten pounds). The Buffer Zone would be slow, but it would be persistent. Using time as our ally, The Buffer Zone would defeat fat, but it would be in the long run.

Back to the scale. While the five-day moving average was helpful to find my true weight, I figured a ten-day moving average was even more precise. I noticed also that, given any ten-day time period, when a low-weight number showed up, even if it was followed by a bounce-up number the next day, it would eventually come true in the moving averages. While using regression analysis helped me calculate my true weight, it was very inconvenient to do the math every day. Then I had another "aha" moment. I couldn't be the first guy to realize that the scale weight had only a 10 percent accuracy rate! Certainly, there had to be someone out there who designed an app that could convert my daily weight numbers into my true weight instantaneously. And you know what? I was right!

A brilliant man by the name of Russ Shanahan over the course of four and a half years (nights and weekends) developed an exponential moving average algorithm to convert your scale weight into your true weight. In a word, it's *genius*! I've been so blessed along this journey to always have the right person fall perfectly into my life at exactly the right time to get to where I am now. Russ's hard work paid off with the creation of the Happy Scale app. With it, anyone can just enter their scale weight and in less than half a second you see your true weight along with a beautiful graph to show you where you are trending.

With the Happy Scale app, Fitstar for working out, my meal plan, and the Buffer Zone, I began.

7/14 BZ 4×4 Month 1 (November 2015)

There are four main categories that have to be balanced if we want to be healthy: (1) the environments in which we place ourselves, (2) the exercise we give our bodies, (3) our sleep, and (4) our diet. Removing clutter and lost time from our environments/relationships, exercising a minimum of ten minutes of strength training a day and thirty minutes of cardio, getting at least seven hours of sleep a night, and following a healthy diet.

I'm amazed at how many "health-conscious" people I meet who are overweight. I'll walk into Whole Foods and see as many overweight people as I do at McDonald's. Our problem isn't that we aren't eating healthy food, our problem is *we are eating too much food in general*. Sure, many of us are junk food addicts, but there are just as many people who are eating too much healthy food. We can all think of many wealthy celebrities that have the capability to have their own chefs cook nothing but healthy food for them but clearly they remain weight challenged. Too much of anything, including healthy food, is bad for you.

If we move the letters around of each category we can spell the acronym SEED—Sleep, Environment, Exercise, Diet. The SEED to good health starts with a balance in all four categories. If we assume you SEE (Sleep, Environment, Exercise) where we are going and have the first three categories in place, we can focus on our Diet, the Buffer Zone Diet. If you look at what I was really changing in my life with the Buffer Zone, it came down to four things:

1. Stop running my diet on just-in food and use a mix, including fat fuel. I was starting off with a mix of 80 percent just-in fuel and 20 percent fat fuel by making sure the time period between my last meal of today and my first meal of the day tomorrow was always 14.8 hours. Subtract 10 hours to get maximum fat-fuel burning and I'd get 4.8 a day or 33.6 hours a week, exactly 80 percent glycogen fuel (just-in food) and 20 percent triglycerides (fat fuel).

2. I abandoned snacks. I saw that they served no purpose except to make me hungry. This was going to be my biggest obstacle. I loved my late-night ice cream. I had stuck to an old rule of stopping my eating three hours before I went to sleep, but all this caused was me having a huge snack every night at eight o'clock. After my full-tank dinners, I had to accept I was done eating for the night. My dad told me he likes to brush his teeth and floss after he's done eating for the day to drive home his commitment. Not a bad idea!

3. I no longer was having three big meals a day but just one yummy, delicious one and two primer meals (300 calories of less) to keep a decent flow

of nutrients directly in my bloodstream at least every five hours. I call that one great big meal a day the Full-Tank Meal.

4. I would front-load all my full-tank meals with a salad and a full glass of ice water to reduce second or third helpings of my favorite foods. I like to call the salads I eat Rainbow Salads because I like to have as many colors of the rainbow in my salad as possible. Dark mixed greens to acquire chlorophyll, Vitamin A, Vitamin C, Vitamin K, and folate to help lower my cancer risks and improve my vision. Orange and yellow fruits and vegetables to get carotenoids that improve my immune function and lower heart disease, get more vision help, more cancer prevention, and more Vitamin A from beta-carotene. Then tan and brown fruits and vegetables to get polyphenol compounds with antioxidant properties to also lower the risk of heart disease and cancer as well as lowering high blood pressure and high cholesterol. And blue, red, and purple fruits and vegetables to grab anthocyanins and lycopene. Anthocyanins have antioxidant properties that help limit damage caused to your cells by free radicals. Blue, red, and purple fruits and vegetables also lower the risk of heart disease, stroke, cancer, macular degeneration, and memory problems.

Compounds from these wonder fruits and vegetables also boost your immune system and limit risk of urinary tract infections.

Of course, I don't expect anyone to remember all this, but it is easy to remember Rainbow Salad. The more colors of the rainbow you can have in your big three-to-four-cup salad, the better!

So, the four main categories to stay centered are: *Sleep, Environment, Exercise,* and *Diet* (SEED); and the four guidelines to follow for the diet are *Fuel mix, Forget snacks, Front-load,* and *Full-tank meals* (The Four Fs). We will refer to these two categories as the 4×4.

In summary: The 7/14 (7 full-tank meals/14 primer meals) BZ (Buffer Zone) and 4×4 (SEED and the Four Fs).

Week 1 Results:

Date	Scale Weight	True Weight
Sunday, November 1	216	215.2
Monday, November 2	215.8	215.3
Tuesday, November 3	213.8	215.1
Wednesday, November 4	213.4	214.9
Thursday, November 5	213.4	214.7
Friday, November 6	212.4	214.4
Saturday, November 7	212.2	214.0

At the end of Week 1, the scale told me I had lost 3.8 pounds but my true weight loss was nowhere near that and the Happy Scale app was there to temper my enthusiasm. My true weight loss for the week was 1.2 pounds. The algorithm had calculated on Day One that my true weight wasn't 216 but 215.2 (I was retaining fluid). Since I'd been using the app since October 24, 2014, the app had plenty of data to determine my true weight. (Note: When you start using the Happy Scale app for the first time, the computer will assign your true weight and your scale weight as the same. From that point on, it will take 10 percent of your new weight and 90 percent of your previous true weight to assign a new daily true weight. I found it takes about a week's worth of weigh-ins to establish a fairly accurate true weight.)

So even though the scale said I lost 3.8 pounds, only 1.2 pounds of it was body fat. The rest was just water. Since glycogen stores are the first reserve fuel tanks that are used and since glycogen is approximately 75 percent water and 25 percent glucose, most diets have great initial weight-loss numbers. We aren't on the Buffer Zone to lose water; we are on this diet to lose unhealthy body fat. Thank goodness we have the right tools to measure our progress.

Week 2 Results

Date	Scale Weight	True Weight
Sunday, November 8	212.6	213.7
Monday, November 9	214.0	213.5
Tuesday, November 10	211.8	213.1
Wednesday, November 11	211.6	212.7
Thursday, November 12	211.4	212.3
Friday, November 13	210.8	211.9
Saturday, November 14	210.2	211.4

For two weeks, with the exception of November 9, my weight was always lower each day I stepped on the scale. The scale, which had been my enemy, was now my best friend in the world. (Note: Never let an inanimate object be in charge of your happiness. The scale doesn't have any skin in the game. It isn't your best friend and it isn't your enemy. It's a tool that given enough time with the Happy Scale app can help you plot your progress. But I forgot that.)

With the scale giving me "good news" every day, I allowed it to be something it had no business being: I allowed it to determine my happiness. Without knowing it, I was allowing my joy to be determined by a scale that has only a 10 percent accuracy rate. I had no way of knowing that once I dropped my excess water weight that getting daily drops would become rarer. Now, don't get me wrong, I did take my daily weigh-ins with a grain of salt since my true weight seemed to lag behind what the scale told me. But I wanted to believe the scale weight because it made me feel good. We are all like that; we would much rather believe a beautiful lie than accept an ugly truth.

While the scale had been kind to me and even my true weight numbers showed I had lost three and a half pounds during the first two weeks, it was difficult not eating snacks the second I got bored. If I was at work or busy, food didn't cross my mind. But as soon as I was relaxing in front of the TV, seeing pizza, hot wings, burgers, and taco commercials made my mouth salivate. Boredom is a void. But I didn't break, not once! In the last two weeks, I had lost more weight than in the previous twelve months! I was so excited! Who knew I was only one day away from it all being taken away.

The Crash

Saturday, November 14, after my weigh-in, I hopped aboard a plane to New York for business for a few days. I was well aware of the effects on the body from plane travel. For starters, the air on the plane is very dry and deadens your taste buds. Perceptions of salty and sweet drop over 30 percent at high altitude. Throw in a cabin pressure that is pressurized to approximately 8,000-foot elevation on the planet and I knew my body wouldn't like that environmental change, even if it was just for a few hours. I did my best to drink plenty of water on the plane to keep my skin from drying out and got up to walk around every hour so blood wouldn't pool in my legs and feet.

Once I got to New York, I stuck rigidly to my Buffer Zone plan. I woke up at the same time each day, worked out, and had my two primers and one full-tank meal a day. Since some of my full-tank meals were later at night, I still kept fourteen hours and forty-eight minutes between my last meal of each day and the first meal of the next day. The result was later primer breakfasts and lunches. If lunch was my big meal of the day when I was in New York, I'd have a primer dinner. By Tuesday afternoon I'd finish my work in New York and head home. Nothing makes you appreciate your bed more than being away for a few days. While I was gone, I didn't have access to a scale so I was anxious to see what I weighed. It had been four days since I was on a scale and I was hoping I'd lose maybe another half a pound. Remember, the scale was my new "friend" and it hadn't been mean to me since I started the Buffer Zone.

D-Day

On Wednesday, November 18, at 8:05 a.m. and only eight days from Thanksgiving, I snuck up and gently stepped on the scale . . . 216.2!!! Oh my God!!! I jumped off. My heart was racing; I was starting to perspire. "It can't be! It can't be!" I said out loud. I picked up the scale and moved it to another place on the floor (silly, I know). Maybe the floor was magically uneven or the gravitational pull on Earth changed and no one told me. I weighed myself three times; twice it read 216.2 and once 216.4. I stopped measuring. All of my two and a half weeks of hard work down the drain!

What a fool I had been. Come on, did I really think I'd come up with the cure to weight loss? Who was I kidding? I felt defeated. Then, all I could think about was food! I thought, "I know, if I'm going to be fat, then I'm going to be really fat! I'll go downstairs and have a huge omelet with tons of cheese and sausage. And then I'll cook four, five—no six—slices of bacon! Yum!" My mouth started watering. "Oh! And a big glass of fattening orange juice! Yeah! Oh, oh . . . and some cinnamon buns!" I felt sure the Pillsbury Doughboy had some in my fridge! I put on my robe and started heading downstairs to feed my sorrows, when I looked over and noticed the Happy Scale app was still on. I hadn't entered my scale weight yet. I paused and thought, "Wait, the scale weight is only 10 percent accurate; what is my true weight?" I entered 216.2 in the app and it said my true weight was 211.3, down .1 from my previous true weight! I wasn't really fat again? Could this all be nothing but water? I'd have to wait an entire day to find out. So, I cancelled the three-thousand-calorie breakfast I was planning and had my primer breakfast. Tomorrow I would find out the truth.

The Verdict

I can't honestly tell you how I felt waiting a whole day to see what the scale would say. I also wasn't sure what I would do if it turned out that the Happy Scale was wrong and I really had gained all the weight back. I knew that a pound was 3,500 calories (I hadn't eaten an extra ten-thousand-plus calories) so I felt the scale had to be wrong but I was still unsure. When Thursday morning came, I took a deep breath, let it out, and stepped on the scale. I was 214.6 and my true weight was up 0.2 to 211.5. It was getting better and the next day would be even better than the last when I weighed 211.2 and my true weight dropped to 211.4. By Thanksgiving morning, the scale had me at 209.8 and my true weight at 210.1! I'd lost another one and a half pounds! With just four days left in November, I was down five pounds!

This one incident taught me a valuable lesson; I almost let one random fluctuation on the scale jeopardize everything I was doing. What's the old saying? "It's not how many times you get knocked down, it's how many times you get up." I think because I had met so much disappointment when I retried the *Men's Health* Diet, I had a short fuse. Sometimes it's hard to remember that the mighty oak tree comes from a single acorn that made good. I knew the scale wasn't accurate and I knew how to calculate my true weight, but when data showed up that made me rethink my beliefs, I got scared.

Sadly, fear more than anything else in the world is the number one cause of weight gain. Fear of not being accepted, fear of failure, fear of not being loved. All of us are worthy of love because we all came from love. I didn't know where the Buffer Zone was going to take me but I knew I wouldn't let fear take control. I would trust in love and follow my heart. Science was on my side and I had to see this through. But short-term, I had little speed bumps to get over. There were four days left in November and I had to navigate Thanksgiving, a holiday devoted to food.

Turkey Day

If there was one time in the year I would typically let the reins go, it was Thanksgiving. I didn't just have *one* Thanksgiving, I'd have five! There was the Big Feast with the family, usually around one in the afternoon, followed by football/food coma and then round two for dinner. All the food (dressing, turkey, cranberry sauce, mac and cheese, ham, gravy, green bean casserole) would be pulled back out of the fridge and we'd all go again. While the food was warming up, I'd take some of the Hawaiian bread rolls and slap some honey glazed ham in them to gobble down as an appetizer.

This of course doesn't count the pumpkin pie, apple pie, and the other myriad of delectables for the sweet tooth. So to recap: two big turkey meals on Thanksgiving Day, then leftovers for Friday, Saturday, and Sunday for a total of five turkey meals!

Clearly, I couldn't do that. But I certainly wasn't going to be the guy who grabs a salad plate and sprinkles a little bit of turkey and dressing and calls it a day. You can't be the guy on a diet on turkey day! My compromise? One big plate. No second helpings, no leftovers. I'd have one full-tank meal with the family, then primer for dinner. Then Friday, back to the Buffer Zone with regular food.

On Friday morning when I stepped on the scale I was 2.4 pounds heavier, but I didn't panic. Yes, I probably had three to four thousand calories the day before but it was just one meal. By the way, the average number of calories consumed in the United States on Thanksgiving is 4,500. For the next few days my weight bounced around on the scale while my true weight stayed steady at 210.1. I made it through Thanksgiving. I hadn't lost any additional weight but I also didn't gain any. I'd take a draw. Month One was over and I lost five pounds. It felt good. Now it was time to move on to December and not let Christmas take me off course. Little did I know what December 2015 would bring.

- The *dots* in the graph on the following page represent my *scale weight* on any given day.

- The *trend line* represents what my *true weight* was for the same time period.

- The *space above the trend line* shows where my *true weight* was at the same time in the **previous month**. The thicker the shaded space, the more weight I had lost over the last month.

FRED CUELLAR'S WEIGHT: NOVEMBER 2015

Best Weigh-In: 209.2 (Down 3.4)
Moving Average: Down 5 in 30 days

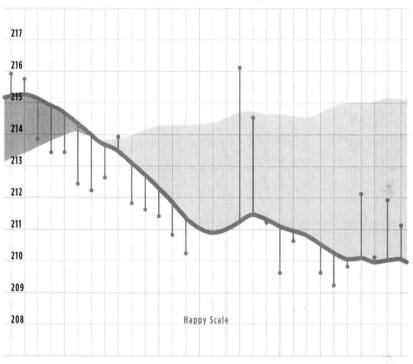

- The *space below the trend line* represents any weight gain from the previous month.

- *Best Weigh-In* represents my best scale weight number and loss in pounds strictly based on the scale.

- *My Moving Average* represents my total weight loss based on my *true weight* on any given month.

Date	Recorded	True Weight
11-01-2015	216 lbs.	215.2 lbs.
11-02-2015	215.8 lbs.	215.3 lbs.
11-03-2015	213.8 lbs.	215.1 lbs.
11-04-2015	213.4 lbs.	214.9 lbs.
11-05-2015	213.4 lbs.	214.7 lbs.
11-06-2015	212.4 lbs.	214.4 lbs.
11-07-2015	212.2 lbs.	214 lbs.
11-08-2015	212.6 lbs.	213.7 lbs.
11-09-2015	214 lbs.	213.5 lbs.
11-10-2015	211.8 lbs.	213.1 lbs.
11-11-2015	211.6 lbs.	212.7 lbs.
11-12-2015	211.4 lbs.	212.3 lbs.
11-13-2015	210.8 lbs.	211.9 lbs.
11-14-2015	210.2 lbs.	211.4 lbs.
11-18-2015	216.2 lbs.	211.3 lbs.
11-19-2015	214.6 lbs.	211.5 lbs.
11-20-2015	211.2 lbs.	211.4 lbs.
11-21-2015	209.6 lbs.	211.1 lbs.
11-22-2015	210.6 lbs.	211 lbs.
11-23-2015	210.8 lbs.	210.8 lbs.
11-24-2015	209.6 lbs.	210.6 lbs.
11-25-2015	209.2 lbs.	210.3 lbs.
11-26-2015	209.8 lbs.	210.1 lbs.
11-27-2015	212.2 lbs.	210.1 lbs.
11-28-2015	210.2 lbs.	210 lbs.
11-29-2015	212 lbs.	210 lbs.
11-30-2015	211.2 lbs.	210.1 lbs.

7/14 BZ 4×4 Month 2 (December 2015)

Since I spent most of my career in the diamond business, the Christmas season had become a busy time. I'd wake up, work out, eat, and run to work. Typically, I would have my primer for lunch at work and then come home for dinner for my full-tank meal. Then, like Groundhog Day, I'd wake up and repeat it all again the next day.

By the end of the first week in December, I was down another pound; the Buffer Zone was working great but my environment was becoming more and more unstable. Teace's dad had to come live with us because he needed around-the-clock care. Teace's mom had been in and out of the hospital, first with a case of pneumonia and then with a heart attack and a series of small strokes. We could all feel the strain being placed on our family when uncertainty rode into town.

Attenuation

In physics, *attenuation* is the gradual loss in intensity of any kind of signal through a system. An earthquake is a good example; at the epicenter of an earthquake the seismic waves are the strongest and then weaken as they move further away. Fat attenuates us. It slows us down, blunts our progress, and cripples our desires. Fat is deliberate as it attempts to diminish and dilute our soul. And yet, I was finally winning the war on fat; I was averaging about a pound of weight loss a week. The Buffer Zone was becoming second nature to me, but like it usually happens, real life takes over while you're making plans to do something else.

After a heroic struggle with a variety of illnesses, Teace's mom, Maxine Prawl, passed away on Christmas Day. Time stood still; everything else was a blur. December came to an end.

FRED CUELLAR'S WEIGHT: DECEMBER 2015

Best Weigh-In: 204.6 (Down 4.6)
Moving Average: Down 4.2 in 31 days

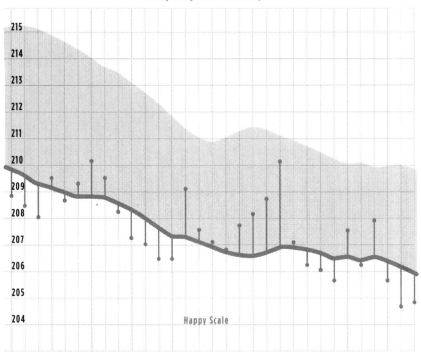

- The *dots* in the graph represent my *scale weight* on any given day.

- The *trend line* represents what my *true weight* was for the same time period.

- The *space above the trend line* shows where my *true weight* was at the same time in the **previous month**. The thicker the shaded space, the more weight I had lost over the last month.

- The *space below the trend line* represents any weight gain from the previous month.

- *Best Weigh-In* represents my best scale-weight number and loss in pounds strictly based on the scale.

- My *Moving Average* represents my total weight loss based on my *true weight* on any given month.

Date	Recorded	True Weight
12-01-2015	208.8 lbs.	209.9 lbs.
12-02-2015	208.4 lbs.	209.6 lbs.
12-03-2015	208 lbs.	209.3 lbs.
12-04-2015	209.6 lbs.	209.2 lbs.
12-05-2015	208.6 lbs.	209 lbs.
12-06-2015	209.4 lbs.	208.8 lbs.
12-07-2015	210.2 lbs.	208.8 lbs.
12-08-2015	209.6 lbs.	208.8 lbs.
12-09-2015	208.2 lbs.	208.6 lbs.
12-10-2015	207.2 lbs.	208.3 lbs.
12-11-2015	207 lbs.	208 lbs.
12-12-2015	206.4 lbs.	207.7 lbs.
12-13-2015	206.4 lbs.	207.3 lbs.
12-14-2015	209.2 lbs.	207.3 lbs.
12-15-2015	207.6 lbs.	207.1 lbs.
12-16-2015	207.2 lbs.	206.9 lbs.
12-17-2015	206.8 lbs.	206.7 lbs.
12-18-2015	207.8 lbs.	206.6 lbs.
12-19-2015	208.2 lbs.	206.6 lbs.
12-20-2015	208.8 lbs.	206.7 lbs.

12-21-2015	210.2 lbs.	206.9 lbs.
12-22-2015	207 lbs.	206.9 lbs.
12-23-2015	206.2 lbs.	206.8 lbs.
12-24-2015	206 lbs.	206.7 lbs.
12-25-2015	205.6 lbs.	206.5 lbs.
12-26-2015	207.6 lbs.	206.5 lbs.
12-27-2015	206.2 lbs.	206.4 lbs.
12-28-2015	208 lbs.	206.5 lbs.
12-29-2015	205.6 lbs.	206.4 lbs.
12-30-2015	204.6 lbs.	206.2 lbs.
12-31-2015	204.8 lbs.	205.9 lbs.

CHAPTER 10

Guinea Pig, Part 2

When I was a kid, my mom read me a story about a little chick who becomes concerned when an acorn falls on his head. Chicken Little ran around telling anyone who would listen that the sky was falling. She convinces Cocky Locky, Ducky Lucky, Goosey Loosey, Gander Lander, and Turkey Lurkey that they were in dire trouble! In one version of the story, the fox invites them all into his lair and gobbles them all up. The moral of that version is be wary of everything you're told and don't jump to conclusions. In the happy-ending version, Cocky Locky warns Chicken Little and the others that they are in danger, not from the sky falling but from the cunning fox that wants to eat them for dinner (clearly a full-tank meal). We learn in the happy-ending version that we have to be brave when things happen that we don't understand and to have the courage to see things through.

In everyone's life a little sky falls. Sometimes it's an acorn, sometimes it's the whole tree. But one thing I can say for sure is that no matter what we do, the day will come when we will meet our fox (maker) and somebody will have a nice dinner. Nobody gets out alive. We must do our best and let our values guide us and not let our environment or others allow us to stray off course. At one time or another we will all have to deal with being fired, divorce, loss of a loved one, depression, sadness, and change. I don't think there is anything that scares more people than change.

The acorn that fell to the ground wasn't looking to scare Chicken Little, it was just hoping to find some fertile ground to grow and reach its potential. It's what we all hope to do—be the acorn that worked with its environment to try to be the best it could be. There will be countless events that occur in our lives to give us pause and a reason to quit. Quit love, quit our jobs, quit life, quit our diets. We can't allow the forces we have no control over to have control over us. Like the sailboat that uses the wind to guide it to new adventures, we must use adversity to harness our inner strength. Food isn't our enemy but it isn't our friend, either. It's a tool that, if used correctly, can allow us to take care of the greatest thing we will ever own: our bodies.

Life is always throwing us curveballs, but if we pay attention, there is always something we can learn from any experience we go through. Will we be defined by our circumstances or will we define ourselves in spite of them? When you read between the lines you will always find the lesson you've been looking for.

7/10 BZ 4×4 (January 2016)

When I looked at every weigh-in number on Monday and compared it to Sunday's weigh-in number, I almost always weighed more on Monday morning than I did on Sunday morning. When I compared my Saturday weigh-in numbers to my Monday weigh-in numbers, I *always* weighed more on Monday than the previous Saturday. One hundred percent! Most of my progress that I was making Monday through Friday was being negated by my lack of work/play on the weekends and, obviously, my overconsumption of food. Moving less, eating out at restaurants more, and probably having too many calories, too. What was interesting is that even in my "take two steps forward and one step back" approach to managing my health, the Buffer Zone was still clearly working. The question was if it could work better. When I say I'm sloth-like when I get home from work and over the weekend, it's not an overstatement.

Also, I realized that Saturday was the number one day people packed on the most pounds in a week. Heck, they should call it Fatter-Day! Understanding the weekends would be more challenging, I put a different action plan into effect. I'd increase my Buffer Zone hours by eliminating my primer meals on the weekend. I would keep my regular schedule of primer breakfast, primer lunch, and full-tank meal dinner Monday through Friday, but I'd switch to just full-tank meals on the weekend to counter the fact I was moving less. I'd make my big full-tank meal lunch on Saturday and Sunday and skip breakfast primer and dinner primer. By doing this, I figured I'd be able to raise my fat fuel burning time. I already was placing my overnight buffer at 14.8 hours (finished eating dinner at 6:00 p.m. and didn't have breakfast until 8:48 a.m.). Since it takes ten full hours to access fat fuel, I was burning 4.8 hours of fat seven days a week. I'd be keeping that up but just Monday–Tuesday (4.8); Tuesday–Wednesday (4.8); Wednesday–Thursday (4.8); Thursday–Friday (4.8); Friday–Saturday noon full-tank meal, no breakfast (8 hours); Saturday–Sunday noon full-tank meal, no primer dinner on Saturday and no primer breakfast on Sunday morning (14 hours); and then Sunday full-tank meal at noon, no dinner primer until breakfast Monday morning (8 hours). I'd be going from 33.6 hours a week burning fat fuel to 49.2 hours! So instead of being on the 80/20 plan—80 percent of my week burning just-in food (glycogen) and 20 percent fat fuel (triglycerides)—I'd be upping my game to 70/30!

I was convinced that by spending 10 percent more time on fat fuel I could be a lot more efficient. The question was, could I handle just eating one big meal a day? I'd never done it before. How would my body react? Would I faint? Feel weak? Speak in tongues? I knew that a lot of diets included entire days where a person only lives on 500 calories (the 5/2 Diet is literally that; eat what you want for five days, starve yourself for two). I knew that wasn't healthy and there are enough testimonials online of people hitting 5/2 Diet plateaus for months. I wasn't going to do anything unhealthy.

The Alternating Diet was an "eat one day, starve the next" diet. That made no sense for a healthy body.

The Warrior Diet starved the body all day and then you could eat anything you wanted all night long, which wasn't a long-term solution.

The *8-Hour Diet* transitioned from no food for sixteen hours (that made sense) but then an eating window of eight hours where you can eat "whatever you want" for as long as you want and as many snacks as you want in that 8-hour window as long as you ate eight particular foods with whatever else you were eating every day. The author describes the eight essential foods as "Power Foods." I found it hard to believe that I could go on an eight-hour binge, eating whatever I wanted, as long as I ate "Power Foods."

The only diet I could find that said it was okay to eat one meal a day was the appropriately named "One Meal a Day Diet." The available research on it showed it was a lousy strategy to lose weight because it didn't allow the dieter to get enough nutrition with only one meal and that the one meal a day would eventually have horrible side effects. A study in the *American Journal of Clinical Nutrition* entitled "Metabolism—Clinical and Experimental" showed dieters had higher blood pressure and blood sugar levels. The *Journal of Inflammation* had a study that one meal a day weakened your immune system. Clearly one meal a day, seven days a week was dangerous. But what about for just two days?

If the 5/2 Diet wasn't killing anybody on two 500-calorie days a week, certainly having over 1,500 calories a day confined to one meal a day on the weekends had to be more nutritious and healthy. The thing is, I didn't know for sure. Could I make up for any nutritional deficiencies I might create with my one full-tank meal allowance per day on Saturday and Sunday with my primers and full-tank meals during the weekdays? Once again, I didn't know. Longer buffer time to burn fat fuel made sense. So, I did what any rational person would do: I tested my theory.

First Big Buffer Day: Saturday, January 2, 2016

When I woke up, I followed my now very ingrained routine: work out, weigh-in, drink eight ounces of chocolate milk. Except now I would skip breakfast. No meal till lunch. While now I know that skipping breakfast is a major no-no, I didn't know it then. By lunch I was famished. I gobbled up my front-loaded salad and then whatever was put in front of me. Usually on Saturdays we would go out to a local burger joint for lunch. When my wife and I were done eating at around one, I knew I wouldn't be having another meal until noon the next day. I was really questioning the concept of a Big Buffer Day, but I stuck to my guns.

When five o'clock came around my mind naturally started thinking of food. This is when I'd normally be having dinner. To stave off my emotional hunger, I drank sixteen ounces of ice cold water. From five o'clock until bedtime, I noticed every single food commercial on television! It's as if the gods were against me! I sipped on more water. By the time I finally fell asleep my dreams were riddled with candy-filled lanes and chocolate glazed donuts. I knew I wouldn't starve, but it took everything I had to not eat that night.

The next morning, interestingly enough, I wasn't hungry, not like the night before. I worked out, skipped the chocolate milk, and then started a countdown till I would get to have my next mouthwatering meal. Of course, before I showered it was weigh-in time and I wasn't sure what to expect. I had not had breakfast or dinner on Saturday so I guess I was expecting to see good news. My Saturday morning weigh-in was 205.6, my Sunday weigh-in was 208.4! Damn! I was up almost three pounds! It didn't make sense. I then reminded myself of the inaccuracy of the scale and looked to see what my true weight was. It was up, too! I went from 205.6 to 205.8. I was not feeling rewarded for my pain and sacrifice. But I had to stay with my plan. By lunch I was famished again and gobbled up my food. Then I went on my Big Buffer Hunger Strike until Monday morning. I won't lie, it was emotionally brutal.

On Monday, January 4, my weight came down a little from Sunday but I was still over two pounds heavier than my Saturday morning weigh-in number. I wasn't happy with my results! I felt like scrapping the whole idea! But I had committed to myself that I would do this for four weekends in a row and I had to stay on course. If by the end of the month I didn't see Monday weigh-in numbers improve, I'd go back to my original 7/14 plan. One of the hardest things when trying anything new is dealing with the failure that precedes success. I remember being a kid and my dad saying "You never heard of 6-Up?" and I would say no. Then he would say, "If they had just hung in there they would have had 7-Up!" I wasn't throwing in the towel yet. I just didn't know the light at the end of the tunnel was a train.

If at First You Don't Succeed . . .

It wasn't until Thursday, January 7, that my weigh-in number was lower than I had started on January 1. The scale said I was two-tenths of a pound lighter but my true weight had briefly dropped then raised up and then returned back to 205.8 pounds. It's frustrating to do your best and not see any difference in your weight after a whole week. The body can be such a fickle thing. Without notice, it can hit a set point where it will retain water to counterbalance any weight loss. Fat gets burned away but water fills the void until it feels comfortable dropping the needless water weight, so many changes occur in the body when it goes through weight loss. When the body loses too much weight it can go into protection mode and trigger inflammation. Inflammation is the body's natural defense mechanism to target any environmental body changes it perceives. Bodies don't like change.

It was entirely possible that even though my scale weight hadn't gone down, maybe I was just a few days away from losing the extra water weight I was retaining. That's how it's possible to be the same weight for days and days, only to find suddenly your body drops a pound or two overnight. Obviously, we just lose a couple of ounces of fat a day and if that void is filled with water, it may take ten to fourteen days for the dam to burst and you see a payoff. It was obvious that I was definitely losing weight during the week and then gaining weight back on the weekend. It just made sense that by cutting out the primers I'd be balancing the scale in my favor.

On Saturday, January 9, I was 203.8 pounds, my lowest scale weight in two years! I so desperately didn't want my weight to hike back up on Sunday. This was my second weekend with Big Buffers. I was skipping breakfast and dinner for Saturday the ninth and Sunday the tenth, so I could hold my weight and not fall backward. My plan seemed sound.

When I got on the scale on January 10, I was almost three pounds heavier! How could I be eating less but gaining weight? What I didn't know then, but I do know now, is that bodies are highly sensitive devices. While I didn't think skipping breakfasts and dinners on weekends was a big deal, I was literally making my body panic. It was that panic that was releasing the stress hormone cortisol into my bloodstream and making my body retain fluid. Fear equals fluid retention. On Monday, just like the weekend before, I lost some of my Sunday gained weight but was still 1.2 pounds heavier than what I weighed two days before. It appeared Big Buffers were a bust. I would keep them up for two more weekends and then go back to my 7/14 plan. Maybe I would just have to live with weekend weight gains.

Positively False

Wikipedia: False Positive Error

A false positive error or, in short, false positive, commonly called a "false alarm" is a result that indicates a given condition has been fulfilled when it actually has not been fulfilled (i.e., erroneously a positive effect has been assumed). In the case of "crying wolf," the condition tested for was "is there a wolf near the herd?" the actual result was that there had not been a wolf near the herd. The shepherd wrongly indicated there was one, by calling "wolf, wolf!"

A false positive error is a type 1 error, where the test is checking a single condition, and results in an affirmative or negative decision usually designated as "true or false".

On Monday, January 18,, my weight was 203.8 pounds, less than my previous weigh-in number on Saturday the sixteenth.

For the first time in two and a half months, my Monday weight did not rise from my Saturday weight. Then on every following Monday from that point on, I would no longer lose ground and gain weight on the weekends. My experiment of ditching primer meals on the weekends and only having one major meal for lunch on Saturday and Sunday finally worked! By the end of January, I was down another 4.7 pounds, followed by 5.9 pounds in February and 7.7 pounds in March.

The 7/10 Buffer Zone was working. Fantastic! It was the Monday to Friday regimen of two primer meals and one full-tank meal and then just one full-tank meal on Saturday and Sunday. I started to wonder how long a good thing like this could last? In so many diets the dieter hits a plateau, and I was sure I'd hit one, too. But, for the most part, the weight was coming off like my hypothesis predicted; slow and steady, about a pound a week.

What I had no way of knowing when I celebrated my birthday in April was that the good times were coming to an end. In my sixth month of the Buffer Zone Diet, I hit my first baby plateau. For the first two weeks in April, I pretty much didn't lose weight and stayed even. I concluded that if dropping primers brought me more success in the past, why not do that again? And with that, I switched from the 7/10 Buffer Zone to the 7/5 Buffer Zone.

I'd have one primer (lunch) Monday through Friday, followed by a full-tank meal for dinner. Then keep full-tank meals for the weekend. By ditching breakfast altogether, it seemed like this would be the easiest way to cut calories and keep going on my road to success. I was totally unaware of the heavy price my body was going to pay for not having breakfast. Sadly, I became more concerned about hitting my goal weight than being healthy. Nutrition took a back seat and vanity drove the car. It's true I had lost a lot of weight, but could I say I was healthy? That would be false. I couldn't see the forest for the trees.

FRED CUELLAR'S WEIGHT: JANUARY 2016

Best Weigh-In: 201.2 (Down 3.4)
Moving Average: Down 4.7 in 31 days

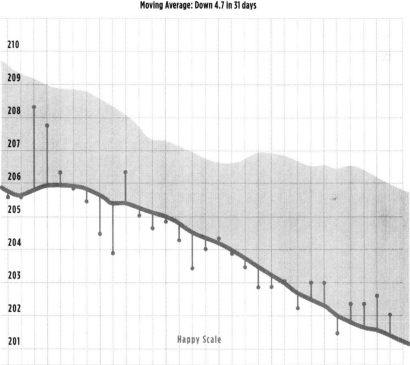

- The *dots* in the graph represent my *scale weight* on any given day.

- The *trend line* represents what my *true weight* was for the same time period.

- The *space above the trend line* shows where my *true weight* was at the same time in the **previous month**. The thicker the shaded space, the more weight I had lost over the last month.

- The *space below the trend line* represents any weight gain from the previous month.

- *Best Weigh-In* represents my best scale-weight number and loss in pounds strictly based on the scale.

- My *Moving Average* represents my total weight loss based on my *true weight* on any given month.

Date	Recorded	True Weight
01-01-2016	205.6 lbs.	205.8 lbs.
01-02-2016	205.6 lbs.	205.6 lbs.
01-03-2016	208.4 lbs.	205.8 lbs.
01-04-2016	207.8 lbs.	205.9 lbs.
01-05-2016	206.4 lbs.	205.9 lbs.
01-06-2016	205.8 lbs.	205.9 lbs.
01-07-2016	205.4 lbs.	205.8 lbs.
01-08-2016	204.4 lbs.	205.6 lbs.
01-09-2016	203.8 lbs.	205.4 lbs.

Date	Recorded	True Weight
01-10-2016	206.4 lbs.	205.4 lbs.
01-11-2016	205 lbs.	205.3 lbs.
01-12-2016	204.6 lbs.	205.1 lbs.
01-13-2016	204.8 lbs.	205 lbs.
01-14-2016	204.2 lbs.	204.8 lbs.
01-15-2016	203.4 lbs.	204.5 lbs.
01-16-2016	204 lbs.	204.3 lbs.
01-17-2016	204.4 lbs.	204.2 lbs.
01-18-2016	203.8 lbs.	204 lbs.
01-19-2016	203.4 lbs.	203.7 lbs.
01-20-2016	202.8 lbs.	203.5 lbs.
01-21-2016	202.8 lbs.	203.2 lbs.
01-22-2016	203 lbs.	203 lbs.
01-23-2016	202.2 lbs.	202.7 lbs.
01-24-2016	203 lbs.	202.5 lbs.
01-25-2016	203 lbs.	202.3 lbs.
01-26-2016	201.4 lbs.	202 lbs.
01-27-2016	202.4 lbs.	201.8 lbs.
01-28-2016	202.4 lbs.	201.6 lbs.
01-29-2016	202.6 lbs.	201.5 lbs.
01-30-2016	202 lbs.	201.4 lbs.
01-31-2016	201.2 lbs.	201.2 lbs.

FRED CUELLAR'S WEIGHT: FEBRUARY 2016

Best Weigh-In: 193.8 (Down 7.4)
Moving Average: Down 5.9 in 29 days

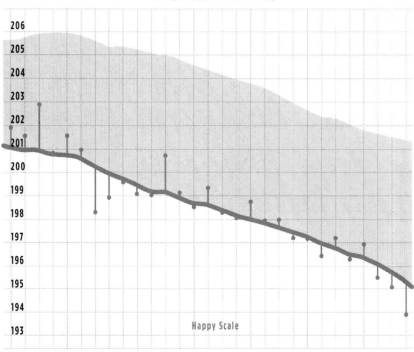

- The *dots* in the graph represent my *scale weight* on any given day.

- The *trend line* represents what my *true weight* was for the same time period.

- The *space above the trend line* shows where my *true weight* was at the same time in the ***previous month***. The thicker the shaded space, the more weight I had lost over the last month.

- The *space below the trend line* represents any weight gain from the previous month.

- *Best Weigh-In* represents my best scale-weight number and loss in pounds strictly based on the scale.

- My *Moving Average* represents my total weight loss based on my *true weight* on any given month.

Date	Recorded	True Weight
02-01-2016	202 lbs.	201.1 lbs.
02-02-2016	201.6 lbs.	201 lbs.
02-03-2016	202 lbs.	200.9 lbs.
02-04-2016	200.8 lbs.	200.7 lbs.
02-05-2016	201.6 lbs.	200.7 lbs.
02-06-2016	201 lbs.	200.6 lbs.
02-07-2016	198.2 lbs.	200.2 lbs.
02-08-2016	198.8 lbs.	199.9 lbs.
02-09-2016	199.6 lbs.	199.7 lbs.
02-10-2016	199 lbs.	199.4 lbs.
02-11-2016	199 lbs.	199.2 lbs.
02-12-2016	200.8 lbs.	199.1 lbs.
02-13-2016	199.2 lbs.	198.9 lbs.
02-14-2016	198.6 lbs.	198.7 lbs.
02-15-2016	199.4 lbs.	198.6 lbs.
02-16-2016	198.2 lbs.	198.4 lbs.
02-17-2016	198 lbs.	198.1 lbs.
02-18-2016	198.8 lbs.	198 lbs.
02-19-2016	198 lbs.	197.8 lbs.
02-20-2016	198 lbs.	197.7 lbs.

Date	Recorded	True Weight
02-21-2016	197.2 lbs.	197.4 lbs.
02-22-2016	197.2 lbs.	197.2 lbs.
02-23-2016	196.4 lbs.	196.9 lbs.
02-24-2016	197.2 lbs.	196.8 lbs.
02-25-2016	196.2 lbs.	196.5 lbs.
02-26-2016	197 lbs.	196.3 lbs.
02-27-2016	195.4 lbs.	196 lbs.
02-28-2016	195 lbs.	195.7 lbs.
02-29-2016	193.8 lbs.	195.3 lbs.

- The *dots* in the graph on the following page represent my *scale weight* on any given day.

- The *trend line* represents what my *true weight* was for the same time period.

- The *space above the trend line* shows where my *true weight* was at the same time in the **previous month**. The thicker the shaded space, the more weight I had lost over the last month.

- The *space below the trend line* represents any weight gain from the previous month.

FRED CUELLAR'S WEIGHT: MARCH 2016

Best Weigh-In: 187.6 (Down 6.2)
Moving Average: Down 7.7 in 31 days

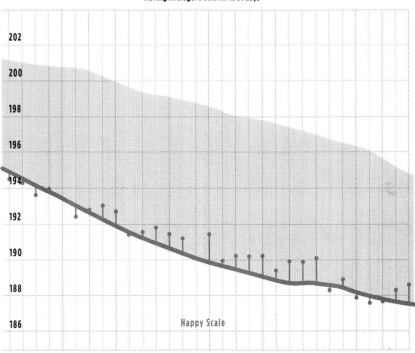

- *Best Weigh-In* represents my best scale-weight number and loss in pounds strictly based on the scale.

- My *Moving Average* represents my total weight loss based on my *true weight* on any given month.

Date	Recorded	True Weight
03-01-2016	194.4 lbs.	194.9 lbs.
03-02-2016	194.2 lbs.	194.5 lbs.
03-03-2016	193.6 lbs.	194.1 lbs.
03-04-2016	194 lbs.	193.8 lbs.
03-05-2016	193.4 lbs.	193.4 lbs.
03-06-2016	192.4 lbs.	193 lbs.
03-07-2016	192.8 lbs.	192.6 lbs.
03-08-2016	193 lbs.	192.3 lbs.
03-09-2016	192.8 lbs.	192 lbs.
03-10-2016	191.4 lbs.	191.6 lbs.
03-11-2016	191.6 lbs.	191.2 lbs.
03-12-2016	191.8 lbs.	190.9 lbs.
03-13-2016	191.4 lbs.	190.6 lbs.
03-14-2016	191.2 lbs.	190.3 lbs.
03-16-2016	191.4 lbs.	189.9 lbs.
03-17-2016	190 lbs.	189.7 lbs.
03-18-2016	190.2 lbs.	189.4 lbs.
03-19-2016	190.2 lbs.	189.2 lbs.
03-20-2016	190.2 lbs.	189.1 lbs.
03-21-2016	189.4 lbs.	188.9 lbs.
03-22-2016	190 lbs.	188.8 lbs.
03-23-2016	190 lbs.	188.7 lbs.
03-24-2016	190.2 lbs.	188.7 lbs.
03-25-2016	188.2 lbs.	188.5 lbs.
03-26-2016	189 lbs.	188.4 lbs.
03-27-2016	187.8 lbs.	188.2 lbs.
03-28-2016	187.6 lbs.	187.9 lbs.
03-29-2016	187.6 lbs.	187.7 lbs.

Date	Recorded	True Weight
03-30-2016	188.4 lbs.	187.6 lbs.
03-31-2016	188.6 lbs.	187.6 lbs.

Head in the Clouds

It was April 15, five and and half months since I started the Buffer Zone, and I was down 30 pounds! I was 8 pounds from my ideal weight of 178 and I could see the finish line! I switched to the 7/5 Buffer Zone and anticipated my plateau would break. I wasn't disappointed. Over the next two weeks I lost 2.7 pounds of the final 8 pounds and by May 16 I lost another 2.2 pounds. Boom! I was down 35 pounds with only 3 to go! I could taste victory. And then, just like the month before, I hit another plateau. Seven long days went by and my scale weight was creeping up. Why would my body quit so close to the end? Would I have to do some more cutting? Would I have to go on the 7/4 or the 7/3 or, God forbid, the 7/0?!

And that's when it hit me. My body was in shock! I was no longer giving my body the right amount of fuel in order for it to operate efficiently. In the last month I noticed I was feeling more lethargic than I had in a while. My workouts were getting harder to accomplish and my mind seemed to be misfiring. I was losing my train of thought, forgetting things to do, and had what seemed like a cold I couldn't kick. I had gone too far. By skipping breakfast, I had not lit my ignition switch each day.

By the time lunch rolled around, I was only eating a primer and not giving my body enough fuel for my daily demands. By the time I got home to have dinner and ate like a king, I practically went into a food coma. I was starving my body when there was work to do and feeding it when it was time to rest. Why was I putting the cart before the horse? In fact, did it really make sense to be having my biggest meal at the end of the day? What if I was fueling myself all wrong? I took out a pencil and wrote out the word dinner. What does dinner even mean? I needed to look it up.

Dinner

Wikipedia: Dinner

Dinner usually refers to the most significant and important meal of the day, which can be the noon or evening meal. However, the term "dinner" can have many different meanings depending on the culture; it may mean a meal of any size eaten at any time of the day. Historically, it referred to the first meal of the day, eaten around noon, and it is still sometimes used for a noontime meal, particularly if it is a large or main meal.

Why was America fat? Why had I been fat? Because we are eating too frequently and at the wrong time. *Breakfast was to get your fire going, dinner was supposed to be for lunch so you could power through your day and supper (evening meal) should be small and light to help you prepare for sleep.* **Snacks just make you fat.** Had I lost a lot of weight? Yes. But I could be healthier. Nightly Buffer Zones (spaces between the last meal today and the first meal of the next day) were critical to get to fat fuel, but *eating the right breakfast to get a jump-start on your day and having dinner at lunch* *were the other two missing ingredients to not just losing weight but keeping it off and being healthy.* **It was time for a new and refined Buffer Zone; it was time to make a change.**

FRED CUELLAR'S WEIGHT: APRIL 2016

Best Weigh-In: 184.6 (Down 3)
Moving Average: Down 3 in 30 days

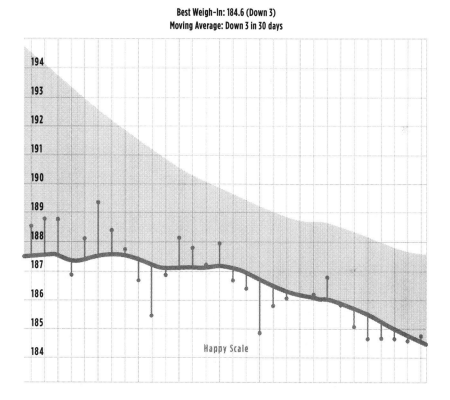

- The *dots* in the graph represent my *scale weight* on any given day.

- The *trend line* represents what my *true weight* was for the same time period.

- The *space above the trend line* shows where my *true weight* was at the same time in the ***previous month***. The thicker the shaded space, the more weight I had lost over the last month.

- The *space below the trend line* represents any weight gain from the previous month.

- *Best Weigh-In* represents my best scale-weight number and loss in pounds strictly based on the scale.

- My *Moving Average* represents my total weight loss based on my *true weight* on any given month.

Date	Recorded	True Weight
04-01-2016	188.6 lbs.	187.5 lbs.
04-02-2016	188.8 lbs.	187.5 lbs.
04-03-2016	188.8 lbs.	187.6 lbs.
04-04-2016	186.8 lbs.	187.4 lbs.
04-05-2016	188.2 lbs.	187.4 lbs.
04-06-2016	189.4 lbs.	187.5 lbs.
04-07-2016	188.4 lbs.	187.6 lbs.
04-08-2016	187.8 lbs.	187.6 lbs.
04-09-2016	186.6 lbs.	187.5 lbs.

Date	Recorded	True Weight
04-10-2016	185.4 lbs.	187.2 lbs.
04-11-2016	186.8 lbs.	187.1 lbs.
04-12-2016	188.2 lbs.	187.2 lbs.
04-13-2016	187.8 lbs.	187.2 lbs.
04-14-2016	187.2 lbs.	187.1 lbs.
04-15-2016	188 lbs.	187.2 lbs.
04-16-2016	186.6 lbs.	187.1 lbs.
04-17-2016	186.4 lbs.	187 lbs.
04-18-2016	184.8 lbs.	186.7 lbs.
04-19-2016	185.8 lbs.	186.5 lbs.
04-20-2016	186 lbs.	186.3 lbs.
04-21-2016	186.2 lbs.	186.2 lbs.
04-22-2016	186.2 lbs.	186.1 lbs.
04-23-2016	186.8 lbs.	186 lbs.
04-24-2016	185.8 lbs.	185.9 lbs.
04-25-2016	185 lbs.	185.7 lbs.
04-26-2016	184.6 lbs.	185.4 lbs.
04-27-2016	184.6 lbs.	185.2 lbs.
04-28-2016	184.6 lbs.	185 lbs.
04-29-2016	184.6 lbs.	184.7 lbs.
04-30-2016	184.8 lbs.	184.6 lbs.

FRED CUELLAR'S WEIGHT: MAY 2016

Best Weigh-In: 179.2 (Down 5.4)
Moving Average: Down 4 in 31 days

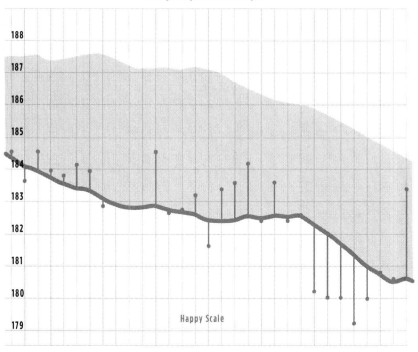

- The *dots* in the graph represent my *scale weight* on any given day.

- The *trend line* represents what my *true weight* was for the same time period.

- The *space above the trend line* shows where my *true weight* was at the same time in the ***previous month***. The thicker the shaded space, the more weight I had lost over the last month.

- The *space below the trend line* represents any weight gain from the previous month.

- *Best Weigh-In* represents my best scale-weight number and loss in pounds strictly based on the scale.

- My *Moving Average* represents my total weight loss based on my *true weight* on any given month.

Date	Recorded	True Weight
05-01-2016	184.6 lbs.	184.4 lbs.
05-02-2016	183.6 lbs.	184.1 lbs.
05-03-2016	184.6 lbs.	183.9 lbs.
05-04-2016	184 lbs.	183.8 lbs.
05-05-2016	183.8 lbs.	183.6 lbs.
05-06-2016	184.2 lbs.	183.4 lbs.
05-07-2016	184 lbs.	183.3 lbs.
05-08-2016	182.8 lbs.	183.1 lbs.
05-12-2016	184.6 lbs.	182.8 lbs.
05-13-2016	182.6 lbs.	182.7 lbs.
05-14-2016	182.8 lbs.	182.6 lbs.
05-15-2016	183.2 lbs.	182.6 lbs.
05-16-2016	181.6 lbs.	182.4 lbs.
05-17-2016	183.4 lbs.	182.4 lbs.
05-18-2016	183.6 lbs.	182.4 lbs.
05-19-2016	184.2 lbs.	182.5 lbs.
05-20-2016	182.4 lbs.	182.5 lbs.
05-21-2016	183.6 lbs.	182.6 lbs.
05-22-2016	182.4 lbs.	182.5 lbs.
05-23-2016	182.6 lbs.	182.5 lbs.
05-24-2016	180.2 lbs.	182.3 lbs.

Date	Recorded	True Weight
05-25-2016	180 lbs.	182 lbs.
05-26-2016	180 lbs.	181.7 lbs.
05-27-2016	179.2 lbs.	181.3 lbs.
05-28-2016	180 lbs.	181 lbs.
05-29-2016	180.8 lbs.	180.7 lbs.
05-30-2016	180.6 lbs.	180.5 lbs.
05-31-2016	183.4 lbs.	180.6 lbs.

FRED CUELLAR'S WEIGHT: JUNE 2016

Best Weigh-In: 176.2 (Down 3)
Moving Average: Down 3 in 30 days

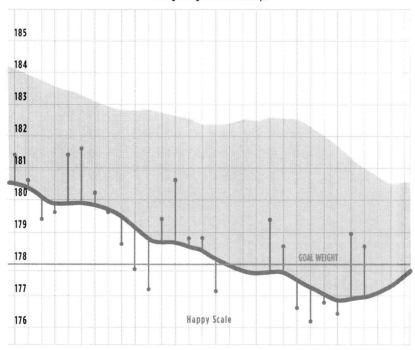

- The *dots* in the graph represent my *scale weight* on any given day.

- The *trend line* represents what my *true weight* was for the same time period.

- The *space above the trend line* shows where my *true weight* was at the same time in the **previous month**. The thicker the shaded space, the more weight I had lost over the last month.

- The *space below the trend line* represents any weight gain from the previous month.

- *Best Weigh-In* represents my best scale-weight number and loss in pounds strictly based on the scale.

- My *Moving Average* represents my total weight loss based on my *true weight* on any given month.

Date	Recorded	True Weight
06-01-2016	181.4 lbs.	180.5 lbs.
06-02-2016	180.6 lbs.	180.3 lbs.
06-03-2016	179.4 lbs.	180.1 lbs.
06-04-2016	179.6 lbs.	179.9 lbs.
06-05-2016	181.4 lbs.	179.9 lbs.
06-06-2016	181.6 lbs.	179.9 lbs.
06-07-2016	180.2 lbs.	179.8 lbs.
06-08-2016	179.6 lbs.	179.7 lbs.
06-09-2016	178.6 lbs.	179.5 lbs.
06-10-2016	177.8 lbs.	179.2 lbs.

Date	Recorded	True Weight
06-11-2016	177.2 lbs.	178.8 lbs.
06-12-2016	179.4 lbs.	178.7 lbs.
06-13-2016	180.6 lbs.	178.7 lbs.
06-14-2016	178.8 lbs.	178.5 lbs.
06-15-2016	178.8 lbs.	178.4 lbs.
06-16-2016	177.2 lbs.	178.1 lbs.
06-20-2016	179.4 lbs.	177.7 lbs.
06-21-2016	178.6 lbs.	177.7 lbs.
06-22-2016	176.6 lbs.	177.5 lbs.
06-23-2016	176.2 lbs.	177.3 lbs.
06-24-2016	176.8 lbs.	177.1 lbs.
06-25-2016	176.4 lbs.	176.8 lbs.
06-26-2016	179 lbs.	176.9 lbs.
06-27-2016	178 lbs.	176.9 lbs.

The Buffer Zones

Within days of refining my Buffer Zone diet, I lost the remaining weight and hit my ideal weight of 178. I discovered through trial and error that there was this envelope in which we can all lose weight. If we could guide ourselves into the right space, our bodies would use fat fuel when we slept and just-in food to work and play. It took me a little over seven months to get my life back and I've been learning a little bit more about myself every day. Intuitively I knew there had to be a way for anybody to enjoy the foods they love and still have a healthy body. I learned that more food doesn't make us more happy, it makes us less.

The Buffer Zone diet was designed so we could have fewer meals that mean more to us. The Buffer Zone teaches us to count meals and not calories. When it was all said and done, I realized there were three main phases to the Buffer Zone for me: the 7/14, 7/11, and 7/7 Buffer Zones. I also learned that once you've gotten all the unwanted fat off, everyone should be on the 7/11 or 7/14 Buffer Zone for daily living.

In Section II, I lay out the three buffer zone phases and how to use them to have your ideal body weight, too. Ready to get started? Just turn the page . . .

SECTION II

Buffer Zone 1 (Your Core)

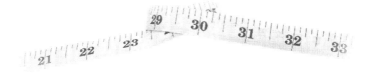

For the sake of argument, let's assume that if you are reading this that you are in a body. I'm well aware that long after I leave this Earth, some being or automaton may stumble across this book and ask "What is a body?" to which I would put it simply, "Everything and even nothing has a container." All things and non-things exist in some environment. If that environment is friendly, your existence is extended; if it is not, your existence is limited. A flower at thirty degrees below zero ceases to be a flower. Environment rules everything. Environment regulates behavior.

But, and here is the question, can we tailor our environment with our behavior so not only our environment is more habitable but also nurtures growth? The answer is yes. If we take care of our bodies (our container, our environment), it will take care of us. When I started this book, I found it interesting that overweight/obese people have three main things in common:

1. In many cases their lives have lost direction and they seem to just be going through the motions. Same stuff, different day. Efficient? But of course! We are a people that get a lot done but we are hardly effective. We aren't doing the right things to move our lives forward. Like a hamster on an exercise wheel, we are moving but not going anywhere.

2. We are overburdened. We schedule every second of our days with little regard for downtime. The candle burnt on both ends is only twice as bright for half as long.

3. We have lost our core, our center. We are out of balance. We work or play until we collapse with little regard for the body we do it in.

There are two sides of the equation to live a happy life: work/play and eat/rest. Eat and rest fuels work and play. It's amazing how much work you can get out of one little calorie. Two thousand calories will allow us to run the typical human body for sixteen hours. Then bodies like to rest. Fueling your body for work/play and not fueling it for rest seems like such a simple proposition to understand, and yet the typical overweight person wakes up in a hurry, doesn't exercise regularly, skips breakfast, has little or no lunch, then arrives home exhausted, ready to crash and fuels up.

We are living life backward. We should be waking up at a regular time each day to not shock the body, be getting at least seven hours of sleep, exercising after our fast from eating, and then breaking our fast with a high-octane breakfast that can raise our metabolism and rev up our engines. The job of breakfast is to get us to lunch. If it is designed correctly, you will have all the energy you will need to keep a positive attitude, clear-thinking mind, and fully-functioning body for five hours. Then lunch takes over; we should have dinner for lunch, meaning lunch should be our biggest meal. The job of lunch is to power us for ten hours, twice that of breakfast.

And what about dinner for dinner? Technically, it's not necessary for the typical person. If your breakfast is designed correctly and if your lunch is designed correctly, the average person doesn't need a third meal of the day. Now notice I said "need." You may "want" a big fancy dinner—heck, you may love eating—but please don't confuse eating as therapy for a success-ful way to do anything but gain weight.

The Buffer Zone recognizes that there is a time to eat and a time not to eat. *If you eat when your body doesn't need the fuel, you will get fat. If you don't eat when your body needs the fuel, you will feel crappy and get sick.* When you eat is as important as what you eat. Not eating (Buffer Zone) is as important as eating.

Let's go over Phase 1, the 7/14 Buffer Zone. You will be on this for the next month to stabilize your body. Then we will move through the other two phases until we remove every ounce of body fat you don't want anymore. This isn't a quick weight loss; this is half a pound to a pound a week of pure fat weight loss. If you're willing to put in the time, I'm willing to give you the road map.

Phase 1: The 7/14 Buffer Zone

Preparation: I've always believed that until you've got a firm grasp of any problem you can't solve it. Our problem isn't fat; our problem is unhappiness. Fat is a byproduct of us eating to feel better; we don't feel good about our lives, so we eat. I can't know what it's like to be you or walk in your shoes. You may have certified proof to justify why you should be allowed to feel unhappy. But where is that going to get you? However horrible you think your life is, it's worse if it's horrible and, on top of that, you are fat. Fat doesn't make the ride easier; it makes it worse.

I may not be able to help you master your job, your marriage, or your life circumstances, but I will teach you how to be a master of your body. If you can't get control of your body, you'll have a difficult time controlling anything that happens to you in your life. The journey we are embarking on has to come with a real commitment to yourself. You have to commit that you will love, honor, and respect the greatest thing you will ever own. Even if you haven't in the past, that ends today. Starting today you will give your body the high-octane fuel it requires, when it requires it, and not flood the engine when it's time to give it a rest. Food is a drug. Know that and respect it. To the degree we love and protect our body, it will love and protect us.

The average person eats two to three main meals a day (a main meal is any meal over 500 calories) and an average of five to seven eating events a day. An eating event is any time you put something with calories in your body.

Our frequency of eating is too high; that has to be adjusted. The average American is eating over five hundred calories of snacks a day. That has to change. Snacks are out. For many Americans, especially women, they eat like birds, four to six small meals a day of only a few hundred calories each. Our goal is fewer meals that mean more to us. We have to trim the thirty-five to seventy eating events a week down to twenty-one. That's right, you figured it out: three eating events a day.

We will be having two types of meals: primer meals and full-tank meals. Primer meals are specifically designed to give you just enough fuel to get you to the next meal. Primer meals are good for a max of five hours. Full-tank meals are good for ten hours. Snacks, like I said before, are eliminated; they serve no purpose except to make us hungrier and keep us eating every couple of hours.

Now before I lay out the eating plan, let's see how much fat you need to lose to be healthy. We have to figure out what your ideal body weight should be using the Hamwi equation.

Hamwi Equation

Women: 100 lbs. for the first five feet of height and five pounds for each additional inch.

> *Example:* A 5'4" woman should weigh 120 lbs.; 100 lbs. for the first 5 feet and 5 pounds for each inch after that (100 lbs. + 20 lbs. = 120 lbs.).

Men: 106 lbs. for the first five feet of height and 6 lbs. for each additional inch.

> *Example:* A 5'10" man should weigh 166 lbs.; 106 lbs. for the first 5 feet and 6 lbs. for each inch after that (106 lbs. + 60 lbs. = 166 lbs.).

Set Your Goal Weight

You now have two choices: you can use the Hamwi equation as your goal weight or you can choose a personal goal. For example, you may think being pleasantly plump is ideal and may just want to lose ten pounds. That's up to you. The important thing is to set a goal and commit to it. If you believe that the goal is too hard or impossible, you may want to break it up. This is your body you are taking back; it's up to you.

We are going to need a way to record our daily weigh-ins. Of course, you can do it old-school with a weight diary (pad and pencil) or use a digital app that can not only record your daily weigh-ins but also graph your progress and give you your true weight. If you read Section 1 of this book, you'll remember that on any given day the scale only has a 10 percent accuracy. Using an app that can calculate your true weight will be a lot easier on your psyche. I use the Happy Scale app to record all my data. I recommend you to do the same.

Month 1 of Your 7/14 Buffer Zone Diet

There are a few questions that need answering so we can lay out your first Buffer Zone week.

1. How many calories should I consume each day?

2. How do I distribute those calories across the three meals I get?

3. What ratio of carbohydrates, proteins, and fats do I consume each day?

4. When should I have each meal?

5. When should I not eat (Buffer Zones)?

6. How much exercise does my body need to get in shape?

7. How do I make sure I get enough sleep?

We will answer these questions in order.

1. *How many calories should I consume each day?*

One of the benefits of the Hamwi equation is that it gives us a baseline for helping us be healthy. Once we know what the ideal weight should be for anyone, we can simply multiply that weight by ten to determine the minimum number of calories that person will need to stay healthy.

> *Example:* The 5'4" woman who should ideally weigh 120 lbs. would require a minimum of 1,200 calories to stay healthy. If she consumes fewer calories, her body will rebel and she will hold on to weight in the form of fat and excess water.

When we multiply someone's ideal weight by ten, we are determining their basal metabolic rate (BMR), the minimum number of calories to keep someone functioning while they may be lying in bed with their eyes open, doing nothing. If a person moves around, we multiply their basal metabolic rate by 1.3 for sedentary, 1.5 for active, and 2 for athletic. The ideal weight of our 5'4" woman is 120 lbs., her BMR is 1,200, her sedentary caloric requirement would be 1,200 × 1.3 (1,560), active 1,200 × 1.5 (1,800) and athletic 1,200 × 2 (2,400).

If you have picked a personal goal weight, different from your ideal weight—say you're 5'4" and are happy to weigh 130 pounds—then you would multiply 130 by 10 to get 1,300 calories, then multiply it by your activity level; sedentary 1,300 × 1.3 (1,690), active 1,300 × 1.5 (1,950), athletic 1,300 × 2 (2,600). The 1,690; 1,950; or 2,600 is the maximum number of calories you can have to hit your goal weight. But don't forget how to determine your BMR. That formula is:

Ideal Weight (Hamwi Equation) x 10 = Basal Metabolic Rate

If you go lower than that your body will not be healthy and you will stop losing weight. So again, for the 5'4" woman, her Hamwi equation weight is 120 pounds and then multiplying it by 10 we get her Basal Metabolic Rate at 1,200. Twelve hundred calories are the least she can have a day and the most is a factor of her personal goal weight times 10, times her activity level.

Example: The 5'4" woman who has a goal weight of 130 lbs. multiplied by 10 multiplied by activity level (let's say sedentary, 1.3) 130 × 10 × 1.3 = 1,690

As long as you stay within your caloric window and eat those calories at the right time, we will be in business.

NEAT

Non-Exercise Activity Thermogenesis (NEAT) is the energy we expend for everything we do with the exception of sleeping. If you are a fidgety person, you may require more calories than just listed. You would only be aware of this if you couldn't maintain your weight and your weight became too low. Solution: Eat more. ☺

---

2. *How do I distribute my daily allotment of calories across the three meals I get?*

For now, you will have two primer meals a day and one full-tank meal. A primer meal is typically 15 to 20 percent of your daily calorie allotment and the full-tank meal is 60 to 70 percent. Remember that primer meals are good for five hours and full-tank meals are good for ten hours. Because of this, it is counterproductive to have a full-tank meal at 8:00 p.m. when you'll be going to bed at eleven. Once you go to sleep, any unused fuel will be stored as fat. That's why it's best to have your dinner for lunch. If you are done eating by 1:00 p.m., you won't be storing any unused fuel.

The idea is to do the best you can to burn up all "just-in food" (food you eat today) to run your body today. Then, allow your fat storage (adipose tissue) to run your body when you sleep (as much as possible). There are three options you have to pick from on the 7/14 Buffer Zone.

1. **7/14 DL Buffer Zone**
2. **7/14 C Buffer Zone**
3. **7/14 D Buffer Zone**

The 7/14 Buffer Zone DL (DL stands for Dinner for Lunch) is the best option and the healthiest for your body. It will allow you to get a delicious big meal right when you need it at around noon to two o'clock. By only having a primer supper (15 to 20 percent of your daily caloric allowance) you don't overwhelm your body with calories when you are ending your day. Fuel up to go! Don't fuel up to sleep.

The 7/14 C (C stands for Combo) means you will have a mix of days where dinner for lunch is possible on some days and dinner for dinner on others. Obviously, the more days you can have dinner for lunch the better. Dinner for dinner loses weight at the slowest pace. It's like taking two steps forward and one step back.

The slowest 7/14 plan is the 7/14 D (D stands for Dinner for Dinner). This means you are having a primer breakfast, primer lunch, and your main meal at the end of the day. You will lose weight on this plan but the results are slower and your body doesn't run as well during waking hours on this plan. It's like having an eight-cylinder car and some of the cylinders won't fire. If you don't give your body the big meal at lunch, your whole system slows down to accommodate less fuel. When you only have a primer lunch, you'll notice that by 2:00 p.m. you will feel an energy slump, followed by a big energy drain between 4:00 and 5:00 p.m. The body and brain are just happier when they get a nice, big fuel delivery at lunch so they can run hard to finish out the day. The more balanced we can keep the body the better.

Don't forget that there are no snacks on the Buffer Zone; high-frequency eating events are what made us all fat in the first place. The hardest thing you will have to get used to isn't having two primers and one big full-tank meal a day, it will be training your mind and body to stop impulse and emotional eating.

Remember (stated in section 1 of the book) the top signs of emotional hunger are:

1. The hunger comes on suddenly. True hunger builds slowly.

2. The hunger is food specific. Donuts, chips, etc. True hunger is not a picky eater. True hunger will eat anything.

3. The hunger compels you to reach for food to change the way you feel (i.e., "I'll feel better/comforted after I eat these Oreos."). True hunger isn't tethered to an emotion.

Anytime we see or smell food our metabolism starts up and you might hear your stomach growl. That doesn't mean you have to eat. Check your watch; a primer meal will sustain you for five hours and a full-tank meal for ten. If it's only been a couple hours since your last meal, you aren't hungry, you just think you are. The days of emotional eating are over. We have to take our bodies back!

3. *What ratio of carbohydrates, proteins, and fats should I consume each day?*

The engine of your body runs most efficiently and smoothly on carbs. You will need 55 percent of your calories in carbs. Cut out the carbs or don't eat enough and your energy level will drop and your mental functioning will suffer. We want to feel good and think well and that's achieved with carbs driving the bus. Twenty-three percent of your calories should come from unsaturated fats and no more than 7 percent from saturated fats. Saturated fats are solid at room temperature. Butter is 60 percent saturated fat. Having just three tablespoons would take you over your daily limit. Only 15 percent of your calories should come from protein. Sadly, the typical American eats twice what they should when it comes to protein. Weight gain, bad breath, overworked kidneys, dehydration, nausea—and the big kicker is, those folks who consistently eat a diet heavy in protein (especially animal fat) are four times as likely to die of cancer. How you balance your plate will balance you.

4. *When should I have each meal?*

Ideally, you should have breakfast within a couple hours of waking up, although that can be extended up to four hours (the 2–4 Hour Rule). While you sleep, your body burns calories at your slowest metabolic rate. The sooner you wake up your metabolism with a healthy primer breakfast, the better. A sedentary person will burn up to a third more calories as soon as they hit the ignition switch and fire up their pilot light with breakfast. When you skip breakfast, your body stays at its slowest metabolic rate that was carried over from sleeping. As long as your body stays in sleep mode, you're going to feel like you're moving in slow motion. Anyone on a normal schedule (wakes up between 5:00 and 7:00 a.m.) would have their breakfast before ten o'clock. If you are a shift worker, just follow the 2–4 Hour Rule for breakfast regardless of when you wake up.

Also, keep in mind that breakfast can be for any meal of the day. Since breakfast will give you enough fuel for five hours (peak performance at three hours and a gentle pull back of fuel between the fourth and fifth hours—the time when the stomach is completely empty and now primed for something more substantial), lunch should be no longer than five hours after eating breakfast. If you don't want to feel any drag at all on the system, eat lunch three hours after breakfast.

Primer lunches will give you another five hours of fuel while a full-tank meal (dinner for lunch) will get you ten hours. The first five hours of full-tank meals are the highest performing hours then followed by a small dip in energy for the hours six, seven, and eight. The ninth and tenth hours of a full-tank meal are only designed for resting and preparing the body to switch to fat fuel as your metabolism drops back to its normal rate (BMR). If you had a primer for lunch, get to your dinner within the five-hour fuel capacity. If you had a full-tank lunch (dinner for lunch) you can delay primer supper (I use the word supper to denote a primer-size dinner) anywhere from five to eight hours after your full-tank lunch.

It's extremely important to keep in mind that the time period between the last meal of the day and breakfast the next morning is the most important time for you to lose excess fat. It takes your body ten hours of not eating anything to allow your body access to adipose tissue (fat). So, if your last meal of the day is seven at night and your breakfast is seven o'clock the next morning, you'd get two hours (12 minus 10 = 2 hours' access to fat fuel) of fat burning.

Since you don't have a lifetime to lose your excess body fat you're going to need to place 14.8 hours between your last meal of the day today and breakfast tomorrow. 4.8 hours is 4 hours and 48 minutes. Four hours and 48 minutes × 7 = 33.6 hours of fat burning a week (33 hours and 36 minutes) which is exactly 20 percent of the available hours in any given week (168 hours are in a week).

Our goal for this first month is to run our body on 80 percent just-in food and 20 percent on old fat fuel. As long as we place 14.8 hours between each dinner and breakfast, stay away from snacks, have only one full-tank meal and two primers a day, the weight will come off! Keep this saying in your mind: Happy Body, Happy Life. We aren't going to shock our bodies into losing weight because our bodies will fight back; we are going to kill our fat with kindness.

5. *When should I not eat?*

It's trite to just say "don't eat between meals," but that's accurate. If you've had a primer meal, you absolutely never eat within three hours after your meal, and if you've had a full-tank meal (60 to 70 percent of your daily caloric allowance) you never eat within five hours after. Primers give you high performance for three hours and then a 10 percent performance drop each hour for the next two hours (20 percent total) and then return your body to its basal metabolic rate (BMR) at five hours. The full-tanks drop off approximately 7 percent each hour after five hours (sixth, seventh, eighth) so that after eight hours your metabolism will also be back at its BMR.

Something to keep in mind: don't eat to go to sleep. Once you nod off, any unused fuel will be stored as fat. Even by some sad set of circumstances you've missed the opportunity for breakfast and ate horribly for lunch, it doesn't give you the right to say, "Oh well, I have a ton of calories I can have for dinner!" No! It's a shame you ran your body on empty all day and for that you probably feel crappy, but you can't eat any full-tank meal that will give you ten hours of energy and then fall asleep in a couple of hours. If it's afterhours and you missed out on meals, it's best to just have a primer supper that will get you energized until bedtime (three hours of energy, two hours of rest) and prepare for sleep. A lot of experts say you shouldn't eat anything three hours before you go to sleep, and they are right. But they are missing the one to two hours your body needs as well to prep for a good night's sleep.

As best as you can, make it a rule:

NO FOOD FOUR TO FIVE HOURS BEFORE LIGHTS OUT!

6. *How much exercise does my body need to get in shape?*

Surprisingly, not as much as you might think. So many people falsely believe that you exercise so you can eat. No. We exercise to stay fit. Your body requires ten minutes a day of strength training and a minimum of thirty minutes a day of cardio. There are countless apps that show you great ten-minute workouts (my favorite is Fitstar) and I usually just hit a treadmill to get my cardio in.

Try to keep your heart rate around 125 beats per minute for a good workout. Obviously, age has a lot to do with your exact range, and if you don't want just a general guideline like 125 to stay alive, I've provided the American Heart Association's recommended target ranges to be healthy in the following chart.

Age	Target HR Zone 50-85%	Avg. Maximum HR 100%
20 years	100–170 BPM	200 BPM
30 years	95–162 BPM	190 BPM
35 years	93–157 BPM	185 BPM
40 years	90–153 BPM	180 BPM
45 years	88–149 BPM	175 BPM
50 years	85–145 BPM	170 BPM
55 years	83–140 BPM	165 BPM
60 years	80–136 BPM	160 BPM
65 years	78–132 BPM	155 BPM
70+ years	75–128 BPM	150 BPM

Apple, Fitbit, Garmin, and countless other fitness trackers can easily be used to help you stay in the zone and keep a healthy heart. My advice is to time your workout as early as possible. When you can combine a charged-up body and a healthy primer breakfast, you'll be raring to go to start your day. Lunch would be my second choice for working out and my last choice would be after work. Since working out revs you up and makes you hungry, I see less benefit to working out and having a big meal and then going to sleep. If you must work out after work, try to only pair a supper (a primer meal that is 15 to 20 percent of daily calorie allowance) with it. That way the big meal and exercise won't make it too hard for you to fall asleep.

Every day the world can throw something different at you and sometimes it's hard to stick to your plans. But if you keep in mind that your body remembers what you do most of the time, you don't have to sweat the few times you get off track. Life is a marathon, not a sprint; pace yourself and don't forget to have fun. Speed kills, endurance prospers.

7. *How do I make sure I get enough sleep?*

According to the National Sleep Foundation, the recommended amount of sleep for an adult eighteen to sixty-four years old is seven to nine hours. For adults sixty-five or older the range is seven to eight hours. The minimum number of hours before we see a drop in physical and cognitive function is six hours for adults age sixteen to sixty-four and five hours for those over sixty-four. Young adults (18–25) that sleep over eleven hours run the same risk of cognitive and physical distress as those who sleep too little. The same goes for adults (26–64) that sleep over ten hours and older adults (65+) that sleep over nine hours; they are blasted with the same mental and physical fog as a sleep-deprived zombie. Too much of a good thing is bad for you and so is too little.

So, how do we get just the right amount? Set a daily start time. Pick a time that you will force yourself out of bed every day whether you have some place to be or not. By training your body to have the same exact wakeup time, seven days a week, you are giving your body the routine it needs to function properly. When we hit snooze buttons, sleep in, nap in the late afternoon, we set up interrupted sleep patterns. Our bodies are a clearing house for memories, muscle growth, and tissue repair when we sleep. Our minds are very active as they consolidate our daily experiences into our long-term memory while our bodies are given the chance to strengthen and restore. Just like an assembly plant, everything has to happen in the right order and just in time if our bodies are going to run smoothly.

Waking up is possibly the most stressful thing you'll do today. Sadly, more people have heart attacks in the morning than at any other time. It's stressful to start a day. Then, just like a car empty on gasoline we wake every day empty on just-in food (food we ate within the last five hours) and need a fill up. Our bodies that have been repairing all night need to be kickstarted. We ignite our metabolism with a one-two punch: Workout and Breakfast. Then we are off! Ideally, we have dinner for lunch and we are guaranteed enough fuel till we hit the sack tonight. Late in the day if we need a little pick-me-up we add supper and then rest, relax, or play—maybe all three.

A good day is a day we prepare for by banking in enough sleep that we can use the following day, then eating before a journey (not afterward) and then thank the heavens for a wonderful day, praying we get another one tomorrow. Want something to be grateful for? Be thankful you're alive.

Typical 7/14 Buffer Zone Plans

Profile 1

Name: Dan Clark

Height: 5'10"

Profession: Stockbroker

Weight: 202 lbs.

Age: 32

Ideal Weight: 166 lbs.

Marital Status: Single

Children: None

Living Arrangements: Condo

Exercise: Not yet

Commute: 15 minutes

Dan's day starts around 6:00 a.m. He gives himself an hour to get up, get ready, either have a bowl of Frosted Flakes or nothing for breakfast, before he heads out at seven. Dan likes to get to work before seven thirty. That gives him two hours before the market opens to get all the research he needs to give to his clients. Dan is in a high-stress business. In order to just make $30K–$40K a year, he needs to manage $10 million in new client assets; seeing he only gets to keep 30 to 40 percent of the 1 percent revenue on those assets under management. Once the market opens, he spends the next few hours calling existing clients to give them recommendations on their portfolios.

Lunch is always short and on the run so he can get some face time with new prospects and then wrap up any loose paperwork. When the market closes at 4:00 p.m., Dan doesn't go home. He spends up to four hours making cold calls, networking, or teaching seminars to prospective clients. Dan is lucky to make it home before 8:00 p.m. on the weekdays. When he arrives home he's exhausted and starving. Dan looks for easy solutions to solve his malaise; he keeps a rack of DiGiorno pizzas in the freezer that can be ready in twenty minutes. Sometimes he doesn't make it home before his appetite gets the best of him and he'll pit stop at Jack in the Box to load up on tacos. Dan joined a gym a few years back and planned to get up an extra hour earlier but that fell through. Then he promised himself he'd start working out at night but he's always too exhausted. Dan is in a vicious cycle of wake up, eat badly, and crash.

His weekends aren't much better; Dan spends six hours on Saturday marketing himself and then surfs the dating apps to see if he can snag a date for Saturday night. Dan veges out on Sunday and on Monday the games begin again.

When Dan was in college he was an athlete on the football team and even played tennis with his mom on weekends. Since he became a stockbroker, it seems his life has been going nowhere fast. Dan is stuck. He feels lousy most of the time and he doesn't know what to do.

Buffer Zone Plan 7/14 DL

If Dan is going to turn his life around, he's going to need to make some big changes, especially with his priorities.

1. Health has to come first, not his job.

2. He's got to schedule his eating plan and then live his life around that, not the other way around.

3. We have to get Dan back on a daily workout routine and cancel the expensive gym membership that he's wasting money on.

4. We will have to change out his sugary breakfast cereal for a powerful primer breakfast that can power him until lunch.

5. We have to switch Dan's big meal of the day to lunch so his body and mind can handle all the stress of his job.

6. We have to teach Dan to grocery shop properly so he can be ready for anything the day throws at him.

7. And finally, we have to schedule a time to unplug from his job so he can regain balance in his life. All work and no play makes Dan a dull boy.

Let's Get Started!

Step 1: Dan has to set a firm, not soft, wakeup time every day. For many of us, hitting the snooze button a few times when the alarm goes off is part of our wakeup routine. We are unaware that those few minutes of extra sleep we steal allow our bodies to begin a new sleep cycle. Then, when our alarm goes off again and again, we fall deeper into a hazy fog. The technical term for it is called sleep inertia; it's defined as a physiological state characterized by a decline in motor dexterity and grogginess after an abrupt awakening. This impaired alertness typically runs three to four hours but might affect you all day. The kneejerk response to mental and physical fatigue is eating because the brain turns to food for a quick pick me up. This wouldn't be so bad except when the fatigue continues we tend to reach for more munchies.

Dan will keep his alarm for six but press himself to immediately get out of bed once it goes off. Dan will keep his wakeups even on weekends and days off. Our bodies are very sensitive and are looking for reliability. By having a set wakeup time that we can stick to 90 percent of the time, we can train our bodies to follow a routine. Bodies love routines and hate uncertainty. We must strive to give our bodies as much routine as we can when it comes to sleep. I could easily make an argument that waking up at the exact same time every day could be the single most important thing you can do for your health. Dan's wakeup time is now a firm 6:00 a.m.

Step 2: After Dan wakes up and goes to the restroom (ten minutes allotted for that), he quickly puts on his workout clothes and does ten minutes of strength training (pick your favorite app). After that, Dan will get in his thirty minutes of cardio. He canceled his gym membership and invested in a treadmill.

After forty minutes of working out, Dan's body is coursing with oxygen from breathing deeply and he's built up a good sweat. The three ingredients to build a fire are oxygen, heat, and fuel. The workout satisfies the first two, and now Dan gets to begin his breakfast, even before he showers and dresses, with 8 ounces of chocolate milk (any protein drink will do). After not eating all night and waking up his body with a good workout, Dan's glycogen stores in his liver and muscles are looking for refueling. The chocolate milk lights the candle on Dan's metabolism and jump-starts his day. Dan's metabolism is now running 33 to 50 percent faster. Dan's got energy! Because it was a protein drink, the energy blast won't last longer than thirty or forty-five minutes so Dan will need to subsidize it with a good primer breakfast.

After Dan has showered, shaved, and dressed, he heads to the kitchen for the most powerful high-octane breakfast he can have: steel-cut oatmeal with fresh berries (blueberries, strawberries, raspberries, blackberries). By seven thirty, Dan is out the door to work. While Dan used to get to work two hours ahead of schedule, he now arrives at work by eight. Dan will realize that working fewer, quality hours is better than working long, less-productive hours. Besides, getting to work full of energy and raring to go beats dragging himself in and just going through the paces.

Step 3: For lunch, Dan has brought a mixed green salad, a sliced apple, chicken salad sandwich on whole grain bread, and a slice of carrot cake. Dan is making a point of having 60 to 70 percent of his calories at lunch (dinner for lunch). By having his biggest meal of the day midday,

Dan has enough energy until he gets home at 8:00 p.m., if he has to.

At around four thirty, after the market closes, Dan can afford a quick primer supper with a couple ounces of turkey jerky, half of an apple, and a small mixed bag of nuts (brazil nuts, walnuts, almonds, cashews). A primer supper of concentrated protein, carbs, and nuts is easy to carry and perfect for a super energy boost to end Dan's day.

A well-designed primer supper keeps you at top performance until you are ready to wind down and prepare to go to sleep. (*Notice:* Dan always gases his car [metabolism] before he makes a demand on it.) ***Fuel to go***, not on the go. If you eat on the run and don't plan your fuel stops, you'll always be behind the power curve.

Step 4: Dan's day revolves around his fill-ups. If we want the time between his meals to be productive, Dan has to make the time to shop at the grocery store. There are key essentials Dan must always have on hand to guarantee he's prepared for anything.

1. Chocolate milk/protein drink for post-workout kick-start

2. Oatmeal, mixed berries, and eggs for designing quick and easy power breakfasts

3. Whole grain bread

4. Apples, nuts, mixed greens

5. Beef jerky, turkey jerky

6. Fresh (low sodium, grass-fed and/or certified organic) deli

7. Fresh vegetables for eating raw or a quick stir-fry

Note: The bioavailability of the nutrients of vegetables is compromised with heat. Translation: You get fewer nutrients from your vegetables if they are overprocessed (heated).

Step 5: The balance of life is work/play on one side of the equation and eat/rest on the other. If we hyper-focus too much of our time on any one of the four elements (work, play, eat, rest) we will be out of balance. If we are out of balance, we won't be healthy.

If Dan truly wants to be successful, he will learn to allot 55 percent of his time to work, 30 percent of his time to eat and rest, and 15 percent of his time to play. Do those numbers sound familiar? 55 percent carbs, 30 percent fats, 15 percent protein. When you stop and take a look around at your life, you'll start to realize that life itself isn't difficult, it's we who make it so. We believe we need so much in this world to be happy when in reality we need very little. We just need each other.

Each day is a small journey, prepare for it. If we are lucky, we will get over 28,000 journeys that will make up our life. Our job isn't to know what will happen, our job is to pack well.

Profile 2

Name: Connie Deroga	**Height:** 5'4"
Profession: Executive Assistant	**Weight:** 161 lbs.
Age: 37	**Ideal Weight:** 120 lbs.
Marital Status: Divorced	**Children:** 2
Living Arrangements: Condo	**Exercise:** Not yet
Commute: 35–40 min	

Connie has to be at work at 8:00 a.m. sharp. Her kids, one and three years old, have to be dropped off at preschool by 7:20 a.m. if she hopes to have a chance to be at work on time. Each morning she has to wake up by 5:30, wake up the kids, feed her little family breakfast, brush everyone's teeth, dress everyone, and get out the door by 6:50 a.m. Connie has eighty minutes each morning to pull off the same magic trick of getting everyone ready to go. This doesn't take into account colds or flus and temper tantrums. Emotions run high every morning. Breakfasts are a mix of eggs, bacon, waffles, toaster strudels, milk, and juice. Connie nibbles on what she makes for her kids but rarely sits down to have a legit breakfast.

After the kids are dropped off, Connie splurges and picks up a Mocha Cookie Crumble Frappuccino from Starbucks and an Iced Caffe Vanilla Frappuccino for her boss. Connie is very good at her job and always seems to anticipate her boss's needs. Connie is the gatekeeper for a bigwig in the oil industry. Making sure her boss wants for nothing leaves her very little time to think of herself.

Connie has no preset lunch hour since she doesn't know what will happen at a moment's notice, but she always keeps an array of nutrition bars and Red Bull to drive her through the day. Connie knows she should do better but her mantra is, "You have to do what you don't want to do so you can get to do what you want to do." She knows she has lousy health habits but that's a problem she will just have to deal with on another day.

The kids remain at preschool until she can pick them up at five forty-five. Every minute she's late she is penalized one dollar. This month alone she's out an extra 253 dollars in late pick-up fees. It seems she's always running behind. By seven o'clock dinner is typically ready with chicken nuggets and grilled cheese as her standby meals, and by eight thirty the kids need to be washed, changed, and put to bed. Once in bed, it's bedtime stories, milk and cookies, and then lights out. Connie typically has to lie down with Evan, her baby, until he falls asleep. Her day becomes her own at nine.

For the next hour, Connie washes clothes, does any kind of precook meal prep for the kids for the next day, pays bills, and then crawls into bed with a small tub of Haagen-Dazs Butter Pecan ice cream. Ten thirty, lights out. Tomorrow, rise and repeat.

How Do We Help Connie?

The first thing Connie has to realize is that no person is an island. She has to ask for help. These are some of the questions that come to mind:

1. Where is her ex? Can he help?

2. Are there other assistants where she works that can work together as a team to cover each other when each of them needs personal time?

3. Would her boss allow the assistants to set up flex schedules where some of the team works 7–4, some 8–5, and some 9–6?

4. Why does she live so far away from her job? Could she relocate to a closer apartment to get some time back?

5. Where's her family? Parents and grandparents can be a huge help in picking up the kids so she can stop incurring late fees.

6. Connie has designed a life for everyone but her. That has to change. Telling her boss she needs a whole lunch hour and working with others at their company are key to getting her life back.

7. Many big companies have day care and Connie may want to consider bringing the kids with her to work. That way when she has a lunch break she could have it with her kids.

As long as Connie feels swamped she will keep putting herself last. Connie has to consider what would happen if she got sick and couldn't work. Her life would collapse. Her health has to be her first priority.

Action Plan: 7/14 C Buffer Zone

Connie realized that in order for her to change her life around, she was going to need to make room for the improvements. It made no sense for her to live so far from work. When she first moved into what is now her old apartment, it was when she was working at Dillard's department store. When she found the better job across town with a big pay increase, it didn't dawn on her to move. It felt easier just to stay where she was and commute. That's now changed with her finding an apartment complex literally in walking distance of her job. There is no wear and tear on her car and her gasoline bill plummeted.

Connie reached out to her coworkers and family for help and everyone was enthusiastic. Her parents loved the idea of spending time with their grandchildren after school. Connie arranged to have them pick up the kids and keep them at their house three times a week so Connie could join a spin class after work. Also with the time Connie is saving on the commute every day, she can slow down a little in the morning and make sure she gets the nutrition she needs to start the day. Connie's new mantra is "If mommy isn't happy, no one is happy."

With Connie focusing back on her health, making more time available during her week, Connie can incorporate the 7/14 combo Buffer Zone. Connie commits to never skipping breakfast and having at least three of her seven full-tank meals at lunch. She's ditched the snacks and does her best to make sure she puts an average of 14.8 hours between her last meal of the day and breakfast the following day. With Connie allowing her body to run on 80 percent just-in food and 20 percent fat fuel,

Connie is well on her way to losing half a pound to one pound a week of body fat.

It's important to remember that our eating habits are a direct response to the stress we are experiencing in the environments we live in each day. No diet will work until we remove some of those stressors from our plate. If we live in an unhealthy environment, we'll have an unhealthy body. We have to make room for ourselves in our own lives. We need space and time to breathe. Remember: you will never be able to truly love or care for anyone until you learn to truly love and care for yourself.

Profile 3

Name: Manny Neilson	**Height:** 5'10"
Profession: Security Systems Owner	**Weight:** 185 lbs.
Age: 51	**Ideal Weight:** 166 lbs.
Marital Status: Married 17 years	**Children:** 1
Living Arrangements: Home	**Exercise:** Not yet
Commute: 1 Hour & 15 Minutes	

Manny's internal alarm clock wakes him at 7:00 a.m. Manny's got exactly fifty-six minutes to catch the train from Westchester County, New York, into the city. In order to be at the loading platform at 7:56 a.m., he must leave his home at seven forty-five and drive to the train. Since Manny values his sleep, he spends every single second he can in bed. Forty-five minutes is just long enough to get up, shower/shave, hug his fifteen-year-old daughter and give his wife of seventeen years a kiss good-bye. There is no time for working out, no time for breakfast.

Once on the train, there are an infinite number of things Manny could do but he only chooses one: he goes back to sleep. (*Note:* Naps over forty minutes lead to Type II Diabetes and high blood pressure)

While at work, Manny is always running around, checking orders, talking to clients, and designing new security systems. Lunch is at two o'clock, and it's typically some high-sodium Asian cuisine. One benefit of Manny's hectic day is he's not a snacker. Manny is a dedicated, hard worker; his mantra is, "Work first, play second." His goal every day is to complete his work so he can catch the 6:45 p.m. train for home. He's successful only 30 percent of the time. If he missed the 6:45 p.m., he would catch the 7:21. Either way, he's not home until after eight and after his wife Donna and his daughter Rachel have long since eaten. Donna usually leaves a plate for him in the fridge. When she doesn't, he scrounges around for something to eat. Dinner is at nine, bedtime at eleven thirty. Over 50 percent of Manny's calories are consumed just a few hours before he turns the light off. Manny spends about thirty minutes a day with his daughter (25 percent of dads spend only thirty-four minutes of undistracted time with their kids a day, while the top quarter spend a little over an hour). Manny is missing critical bonding time with Rachel.

When Manny was dating Donna, they spent over fifteen hours a week together with each other's undivided attention. Their love flourished. Now that they've settled into married life, they're lucky to get twenty minutes a day. Ask someone with a family why they are working so hard and their first response is that they are doing it for their family. Family is number one. How do you think Manny is doing in this category?

In practically every single case I studied of obese people, food had become a substitute for love. The quality of the relationships people had with themselves and others had died on the vine so they self-medicated with food. Run on empty all day, to match our emotions, then knock ourselves into a food coma to sleep.

How do we save Manny and his family? Before we can devise a rescue plan, we need to be crystal clear about where his problems lie. We will use the 4×4 format to target his troubled areas.

SEED (Sleep, Exercise, Environment, Diet)

Sleep: It appears that Manny is getting enough sleep but nothing could be further from the truth. When we look closer at Manny's day we realize that he downs coffee all day in order to keep energized. Studies show that caffeine can affect the quality of your sleep for up to twelve hours after your last cup. Manny also likes to have a nightcap of bourbon with his meal and is staring at some type of bright screen (TV, iPad, home computer) until he goes to sleep. Because his body is dealing with processing a heavy meal, the aftereffects of caffeine consumed late in the day, alcohol, and bright lights that are screwing up his melatonin levels (a high level is required to get a good night's sleep), Manny misses out on the deep sleep his body needs to repair and prepare itself for the next day. Also, Manny is not getting any exercise; therefore, he lowers the likelihood of getting any quality sleep to almost zero.

When Manny is pressed for how he feels on a daily basis, he complains of the following symptoms:

- Fatigue

- Sleepiness

- Morning headaches

- Dozing off at inappropriate times

Exercise: While Manny would argue he doesn't have time to exercise, he doesn't understand the long-term damage he's doing to his body. Manny is aware that he has put on a few pounds since his days of running track in college and running marathons in his twenties, but he's always been able to justify his actions and convince himself that he'll get back on the workout bandwagon soon.

What Manny is unaware of is his blood pressure can lead to heart disease and Type II Diabetes. All because Manny has designed his day around work and not around being healthy. Every task seems to be taking him twice as long. When he makes mistakes, he loses his temper and yells at everyone. If our bodies aren't getting the sleep, exercise, nutrients, and healthy environment they require, our emotions run high. Impatience, anger, doubt, sadness, depression, and anxiety all go through the roof when our bodies are unhappy. Even Manny's bone strength and muscles are atrophying. Manny is a time bomb waiting to go off.

Environment: The quality of our lives is driven by the quality of the relationships we have. Loving relationships with ourselves and others are the only types of environment in which our bodies can grow and prosper. But if we look at Manny's relationship with his exhausted mind and body, as well as the little time he has for his family, we can see that Manny needs a major overhaul and not just in his diet. He has to start getting a good night's sleep. He has to start exercising (ten minutes of strength training and thirty minutes of cardio a day), reconnect with his family, and incorporate his new Buffer Zone.

Diet:

1. Use fat fuel to run his body at least 20 percent of the time.

2. Forget snacks and only have one main meal a day and no more than two primer meals a day (twenty-one eating events each week).

3. Front-load his meals with a healthy salad and/ or vegetables.

4. Have one full-tank meal a day (where 50 to 70 percent of his daily calories are consumed).

Action Plan: 7/14 D Buffer Zone

Life is a funny thing; tell a dying person you have a cure to save his life and he will sell everything he owns to acquire the cure. Tell a "healthy person" (no current signs of disease yet) that for a small price she can improve her health and help prevent horrible diseases, and she will pass it up. We will do more to stop pain than we will do to extend our lives. Why do we have to wait to get sick before we do what we should do to maintain our bodies?

Because Manny loses one hour and fifteen minutes each way in his commute he's going to have to make some major changes in his life if he's going to prevent the catastrophe that awaits him in the future. In order to get his required deep sleep, he will have to stop the caffeine by 10:00 a.m., allowing his body to have the twelve hours it needs to funnel it out of his system. He's going to need to pick a firm wake-up time that he can commit to seven days a week; once he's up, no sleeping on the train. When we take a nap so soon after waking up, it starts another sleep cycle that can take hours to snap out of.

Since Manny is the boss and most of his work is monitoring others, he has to ask himself does he have a competent Number Two person in his organization that he can count on? If he does, he can delay his arrival time by one hour, giving him the time he needs to exercise and have breakfast with his wife. That simple little hour delay can allow his body to get the jump-start he needs to wake up his metabolism and give him the energy to start his day. That way when he gets on the train, he can work—making any necessary phone calls (what he usually does during the first hour of work at the office) and going through emails.

Once he arrives at work, he has accomplished the same work as before and he won't be so listless. One of the other problems that is wrecking his health is eating over 50 percent of his caloric intake just a few hours before going to bed. Don't fuel a car to park it in the garage. So instead of eating that big meal at 9:00 p.m., Manny brings last night's dinner to work with him. In an ideal world, Manny would eat that dinner for lunch but he has the flexibility to eat it before 5:00 p.m. By giving his stomach the five hours it needs to empty, by the time Manny is ready to go to bed all of the heavy digestive lifting will be over and he'll sleep like a baby.

In the past, Manny had heavy, sodium-based, Asian takeout for lunch, but now that Manny has added a primer breakfast, he's going to abandon that for either a primer lunch (have some of his dinner for lunch and save the rest until five) or he can just have something like a fresh turkey sandwich on whole wheat/whole grain bread. By the way, the only way to know if the bread you're eating is healthy is to look at the ingredients list on the bread. If it doesn't list whole wheat or whole grain as one of the first ingredients, it isn't what's best for you.

For Manny to get his life back, he has to fuel up before he starts his day and plan ahead for what he will eat and when. The all-day coffee, morning naps on the train, and no exercise were all zapping Manny's energy. His mantra has to be *fuel to go*, not to stop.

By adding that one hour to his day, Manny will be able to help his sleep and build his body's strength back with exercise. He will still need to make more time for the people he loves. Life can't just be about work. Quality relationships are built on trust, and trust requires constant communication. One other suggestion for Manny would be to consider the possibility of working from home or half days from home. If Manny doesn't invest the time into his family life now, he might wake up wealthy but a lonely old man. Our loved ones are patient and will wait but they won't wait forever. One day, Manny could come home to an empty house.

Love your body, challenge your mind, and help those you love be the greatest version of themselves they can be. And then maybe, when you're old and gray, you'll have someone to snuggle with and say good night to. We have one life. Love and cherish it.

CHAPTER 12

Buffer Zone 2
(Accelerated Fat Burning)

Since 1970, the average American has increased the number of calories he or she consumes by 523 a day. Fifty percent of those calories are from fats and sugars and all of those calories are being consumed in the form of snacks. It's like the old joke where a person declares he is on the "seafood diet," meaning "any food I see, I eat!"

Apparently, we have all been on a "seafood diet." We've been eating two to three main meals a day (only need one) and having five to seven snacks/eating events a day on top of that (all we need are one or two more well-designed primer meals that are each approximately 20 percent of our daily caloric allowance and follows a 55 percent carb, 30 percent fat, and 15 percent protein makeup).

The frequency of our eating is the reason we are obese. When you start to understand that the most any of us needs on a weekly basis for eating events is twenty-one (three a day), NO SNACKS! Then and only then will we bring our health back.

As soon as you've gone four weeks and stuck to no more than seven full-tank meals a week (one a day) and no more than fourteen primer meals a week (two a day) you'll be ready to burn more fat. But if you are still grabbing a chocolate from the receptionist's desk at work, sneaking in chips or Twizzlers from your private stash, then you aren't ready for Buffer Zone 2. Buffer Zone 2 is strictly for people who have built up the tolerance for no snacking. If you've accomplished that, read on. If not, stay with Buffer Zone 1 until you've gone four full weeks without snacking. Let's continue!

After a successful first month on the Buffer Zone, it may have already dawned on you that if you increase the time between your last meal of the day and breakfast the next morning, you'll burn more fat fuel. So how do we do that? Well, we can't skip breakfast, because we have to *fuel to go*. We can't skip lunch (that's ten hours worth of fuel we need to drive us through our day), but what about supper? Hmm . . . supper, believe it or not, is the one and only throw-away meal of the day! Think about it: if you have your full-tank meal at lunch and are done by one o'clock (that's enough fuel to get you until eleven o'clock tonight) why do you "need" a primer supper at five or six o'clock? The short answer is you don't.

If you planned a well-thought-out primer breakfast (fuel to get you going until lunch) and a well-designed, nutritious, full-tank lunch, you have plenty of fuel to get you till bedtime. Nighttime eating is really just a bad habit that serves little or no purpose (from a nutritional, get *fuel to go* standpoint). I'm not saying that dinner or supper with the ones you love isn't important, but what I am saying is fueling up your body with a full-tank meal when you're just going to be going to sleep in a few hours makes no sense. Let me use the following analogy that might hit my point home. Pretend that you had a very unique car, and that no matter how much gas was in it when you parked it in your garage at night, it would always be on empty the next morning.

Furthermore, any gas that was left in the car overnight would add weight to the body of the car and rust. If you kept bringing the car home with a full tank of gas, eventually the car's body would weigh so much that it wouldn't be able to move and get you around. That's exactly what we are doing to the greatest thing we will ever own, our bodies. We are fueling them up to go nowhere at night and starving them of fuel during the day. We have to reverse that. If you've conquered the battle over the snacks, let me introduce you to Buffer Zone 2: Accelerated Fat Burning!

7/11 DL Buffer Zone and 7/11 C Buffer Zone

For the next stage of our weight loss, we are going to ditch three suppers. If you've been on the 7/14 D Buffer Zone, this is going to require you to have your full-tank meal at lunch three times a week at a minimum. The rest of the week you can go back to a primer breakfast, primer lunch, and full-tank dinner.

For those of you that have been on 7/14 Combo and 7/14 DL (dinner for lunch), you'll be eliminating three primer suppers a week. These mostly habit-driven meals will be fairly easy to abandon now that you've mastered the skill of not snacking. On average, you'll pick up an additional five and a half hours a day when you just have a primer breakfast and full-tank dinner for lunch (60 to 80 percent of your daily caloric allowance). So, if we'd already been burning 33.6 hours of fat fuel a week (20 percent of a 168-hour week) we will be burning 50.1 hours of fat fuel instead! That's an increase of almost 50 percent more fat fuel! Boom! We will be going from 80 percent just-in food (glycogen) and 20 percent fat fuel (triglycerides) to 70 percent just-in food (glycogen) and 30 percent fat fuel (triglycerides). Our new 70/30 fuel mix is going to rev up our weight loss and give us a lot more time and energy on our hands.

When I was a habitual night eater (had my biggest meal of the day when I came home from work), the question, "What's for dinner?" was always a problem for my wife and me to deal with every night. Now on the days where we've had our last meal of the day at lunch, we've eliminated that nagging question and are free to do something else with our time that we used to devote to (1) figuring out what we were going to eat, (2) preparing food or going to a restaurant to acquire said food and (3) the time it takes to be seated, order, and eat our dinner. Dinner was easily gobbling up over two hours of our day, every day! That is time that my wife and I can either spend on our hobbies or relaxing.

As a society, we love to "break bread" with the ones we love and none of that has to change. We just have to be more organized about when and where we choose to get together. If we communicate our needs and plan ahead, we can nourish our bodies and forge our relationships with our family and friends.

I'm sure the restaurant industry won't be a big fan of my book at first, but soon they will realize as people's eating habits change and we all become healthier, it will be good for them in the long run. Healthier people live longer and longer-living people will eventually eat more food. Less revenue per day will be balanced out by more days of revenue.

When I think back to how much of my life has been ruled by food, it's crazy. As a child and then continued as an adult, every celebration, every milestone was celebrated with food. Food had slowly but surely been packaged as a reward. Get good grades, go out to dinner. Have a birthday, go out to dinner. Get a promotion, have an anniversary, get dinner, get dinner. Food had also become a security blanket. Feel sad, eat something. Lose a job, break up with a boyfriend or girlfriend, get a divorce, or even get bored and food was there to give us a quick pick-me-up. We have been rewarding and sedating ourselves with food. Food is not our buddy or best friend or our enemy. *Food is fuel.*

As we cut ourselves free from our addiction to food, we will find ourselves with a lot more time on our hands. The question is, what will you do with it? I've always believed that one of the secrets to happiness was personal growth. If I can pick up a book, try a new experience, travel, spend more time with people I love, I grow and prosper. In Buffer Zone 2 you are going to get some of your life back. What are you going to do with your extra time?

The Buffer Zone Diet

The Four Domains

If you stop and think about the one word most Americans fear their physicians telling them, it would be cancer. "You have cancer." No one wants to hear that. In the article written by Aaron E. Carroll entitled "Helpless to Beat Cancer? Actually, Quite a Bit is Under Your Control," Professor Carroll points out the four domains that, if we apply healthy lifestyles in, we can potentially drop our risk of getting cancer by as much as 50 percent! They are: smoking, drinking, obesity, and exercise. The catch is we have to go four for four. Meaning, if you fail in even one of these domains you are putting yourself in the high-risk group of getting cancer.

While getting a perfect score may seem daunting at first, I think you'll come to the same conclusion Professor Carroll came to as well: it's totally doable. In order to get a gold star in the smoking domain, "not smoking" means you've never smoked or quit smoking for the last five years. Even if you are currently smoking and you quit today, you'd be just five years away from potentially cutting your risk in half! Think of it this way: if you were born in 1960 and are a male, there is a 53.5 percent chance you will get cancer in your lifetime and a 47.5 percent if you are a woman, and that's if you don't change your lifestyle one iota.

Imagine you're playing Russian Roulette (and you are) with a .22 revolver being placed to your forehead with nine rounds. If you do nothing to help yourself, it's like leaving five of the nine chambers full and giving it a spin. But if you quit smoking now and clean up your game in the other three domains, we get to remove two to three bullets from the gun! Naturally, there is no way to remove all of the bullets because some things, like age, race, and family genetics, are beyond our control. But doesn't it make sense to remove the bullets that don't have to be in the gun? If you're smoking now, stop.

In the drinking domain, we're not talking about abstinence (of course, unless you have a drinking problem) but applying a moderate alcohol consumption rule. No more than one drink a day on average for women and no more than two drinks a day on average for men.

Now, before you go out and buy a new, larger, single-serving container that can hold an entire bottle of wine, here's what is considered a serving of alcohol:

U.S. Dietary Guidelines for Americans

Beer: 12 ounces

Spirits: 1.5 ounces

Wine: 5 ounces

Also, no binging! Binging destroys your cells. You can't refrain from alcohol all week and then have a bender on Saturday night. Binge drinking is defined as having four or more drinks for a woman and five or more drinks for a man within a two-hour period. In order to make the obesity cut, you have to have adequate weight. That is defined by having a BMI of at least 18.5 and no more than 27.5. Overweight is 25 and obese is 30 or more. No one is looking for absolute perfection, but clearly there has to be personal responsibility here. Hunger can no longer be your master. There is a time to eat and a time not to eat. Just make sure you know what time it is.

The final domain isn't really that hard, either. The minimum amount of exercise to lower your cancer risk is seventy-five minutes of vigorous-intensity activity a week and at least 150 minutes a week of moderate-intensity activity. Imagine again, there is a gun pointed to your head with five live rounds and four empty chambers. Don't you want to take three bullets out of the gun before you pull the trigger?

Typical 7/11 DL Buffer Zone Plan

Profile 4

Name: Ashley Hernandez	**Height:** 5'8"
Profession: Auditing Manager	**Weight:** 154 lbs. (was 160)
Age: 28	**Ideal Weight:** 140 lbs.
Marital Status: Divorced	**Children:** None
Living Arrangements: Townhouse	**Exercise:** Yes
Commute: 25 minutes	

After Ashley graduated from University of Texas–Austin's McCombs School of Business, she was quickly recruited by all Big Four accounting firms and eventually chose EY (formerly Ernst and Young). Ashley has always had a head for numbers and loved the idea of working with multinational corporations. Within five years (right on schedule), she was promoted to audit manager and when everything else continues to go her way, she hopes to be promoted to senior manager in the next two years.

Of course, the big prize of partner is on her radar by the time she is thirty-five—or sooner.

Ashley has always been goal-oriented; she is a leader and was top of her class. That's why it came as a little bit of a shock to her when she suddenly noticed that her clothes were fitting a lot tighter. When she stopped to think about it, she realized that her eating schedule during peak periods (usually January through March; she has quite a few clients in Singapore) was having her working as late as 2:00 a.m. and eating late. In the past, when she put on a few, she'd just hit the gym and the weight would fall off. But now, six years removed from her collegiate days, the weight hadn't gone anywhere. Ashley then went on the 7/14 DL Buffer Zone last month after tax season and has been able to drop six pounds.

Now that Ashley has become a master at ditching the snacks and late-night meals, she feels better than she has for years. Like all of us, Ashley wants to waste as little time as possible and crank up the fat burning. She's decided that during off-peak hours where her schedule runs 9:00 a.m. to 6:00 p.m., she will get in her primer meal and exercise in earlier before work and then have a leisurely long lunch (a privilege of being manager and team leader) where she will get all the nutrients she needs with her front-loaded, full-tank lunch and even dessert.

On paper, it all looks so easy. What she doesn't count on is the unexpected long list of administrative duties that are thrown on her from client billing and chasing after bad debt. Recently she was put in charge of new engagements and staffing the teams (there is an extremely high turnover rate at Big 4 firms). Conceptually the 7/11 Buffer Zone doesn't seem that much harder than the 7/14 DL she had been on before. But as stress at the office mounts and peak periods are on the horizon, Ashley begins a downward spiral she set into motion when she said three little words to herself: "Just this once."

You see, all the girls were going out for margarita night and Sally's brother, who has been described as a "catch" (and single) was going to be there. Ashley's been meaning to get back into the dating pool since her divorce two years prior and thinks this is the perfect opportunity. So she says to herself, "I've been good. I lost over six pounds and I deserve 'just this once' to reward myself." And with that, she enjoys a night of drinking and eating and even a surprise "It's been wonderful to meet you/can't wait to see you again" goodnight kiss from Kevin, Sally's brother. It all goes well until Ashley wakes up the next morning.

As she's about to log in to her Intranet chat portal to review questions her team members have for her, she steps on the scale and sees five pounds of weight gain staring back at her! Ashley screams, jumps off the scale, kicks it, stubs her toe, hops around on one foot until she lands on a loose area rug and then as the rug shoots out from underneath her, she crashes to the floor.

Consequence: Broken toe, sprained ankle, four to six weeks in a restrictive boot.

What Does Ashley Do Now?

They say life is what happens to you when you were busy making other plans. I can attest to the fact that it is painful to see a large weight gain after what seems like a harmless little "cheat" snack meal or day. So much of eating is emotionally tethered; it's hard not to reach for food when times are good or when they've been a little rough. One of Ashley's problems is continuing to see food as a reward. It's ironic that we "reward" ourselves with food for watching what we eat. Two steps forward, one step back. The right mind-set is the key.

Ask yourself this: would I rather get what I want now (craving) or what I want most (being healthy). The reason it's so hard to see the big picture is because instant gratification is, well, so instant. Where choosing healthy is a process, a direction, we never cross the finish line of being healthy and then call it a day. Healthy is a lifestyle. The good news for Ashley is our bodies tend to remember what we do most. And for Ashley, that's being mostly responsible. When Ashley realizes that all the weight gain is water and will take at most a week to come off, she'll feel better. Losing weight is not a linear process, but Ashley (and the rest of us) always has a negative reaction when she sees the scale go up. Look at the stock market; one day it's up, the next it's down. As long as we feed our bodies to start our days, refuel them at midday, and then give our digestive system a break when we rest and sleep, the unhealthy fat does come off.

One of the hard things for Ashley will be getting in her regular physical activity while in a foot brace. This is where creativity will come in. Pilates is a great example of a good mind and body alignment system that can be done by just about anyone in any condition. Healthy bodies are strong bodies, and strong bodies need resistance training if they are going to be resilient.

Here's what Ashley does:

1. She gets back on the horse and back to her 7/11 plan; one front-loaded, full-tank meal a day with two primers on four days of the week and then one breakfast primer with one full-tank meal on the other three days.

2. Do her best to make sure she keeps up her sleep, exercise, and home/work environment. When we fall off the wagon, we tend to jeopardize all areas of our lives. Sleep, exercise, stable environment, and diet are all tied together. Don't let a slip-up in one area get you to slip up in others.

3. While so many diets have "cheat" days and meals, it's best to understand that the Buffer Zone is designed so you can have whatever you want but not whenever you want it. If you can't time your meals accordingly, the Buffer Zone can't work for you.

4. Ashley has to understand that life is filled with lots of special occasions (birthdays, 4th of July, Christmas, etc.) if she knows when she wants to have her big meal of the day (lunch or dinner), choose that. Just don't choose both. Also, the 7/11 Buffer Zone is about getting 30 percent of your 168 hours (fifty or more) in the Buffer Zone a week. If you are short a little one day, make up for it by having lunch a little earlier on another day or even having a later breakfast to add Buffer Zone hours.

There are two reasons why the Buffer Zone works. (1) We eat before we ask our bodies to take us through the day and not after, and (2) we eat food that satisfies our taste buds every day. No diet will become a lifestyle if we aren't satisfied. The key to anything satisfying is having the ability and willingness to wait for what we really want most.

The Powers of Potassium and Sodium

There are two essential nutrients our bodies require to function correctly; they are potassium and sodium. They help regulate blood flow and our fluid levels both inside and outside our cells. If our bodies don't have enough sodium (rarely our problem) we can run into cardiovascular, neurological, and muscular problems. Without enough sodium, our nerve impulses and muscular contractions are out of whack.

Potassium is a counterbalance to sodium, kind of like the yang to the yin of sodium. While sodium allows our cells to maintain fluid levels, potassium allows the cells to remove and break down carbs for usage. Our bodies require only 500 milligrams of sodium a day, yet the typical American consumes over 4,500 milligrams a day! That's nine times our daily requirement! When our body gets inundated with sodium, it is forced to find a way to dilute all that sodium and it does so with retaining water.

The problem? When cells are bloated with water, it makes it harder for your blood to flow, hence high blood pressure. Potassium and sodium are electrolytes that work as conductors in our blood and cellular fluid. They really work together in a symphony of equilibrium. If there is too much sodium in our system, potassium works to flush out the sodium water cocktail so your blood pressure comes down. The body requires 4,700 milligrams of potassium a day to keep our sodium levels in check.

But once again, here we have a problem. Americans are eating nine times the minimum sodium required and twice the 2,300 milligrams considered maximum by the Institute of Medicine (for Americans who already have high blood pressure, are over the age of fifty, or African American, 1,500 milligrams of sodium is maximum). So, one solution to our heavy sodium diet would be to eat more potassium that occurs naturally in foods like bananas, apricots, lima beans, tomatoes, or pretty much all meats.

Over-the-counter supplements don't really help because they carry such small amounts of the mineral. The problem with the "eat more potassium" solution is this: it's hard enough to get your daily requirement of potassium, much less add more to compensate for all the added sodium in our diets from processed foods and salt shakers. One large banana would only give you 10 percent of your daily allotment. Because Americans aren't getting enough fruits and vegetables a day, they aren't even coming close to balancing the sodium/potassium scale. And they are paying for it with fatigue, constipation, muscle weakness, and even abnormal heart rhythms.

So, what's the real solution? Of course, eat more fruits and vegetables (I've added a banana a day to my diet) but that won't be enough. Stop adding salt and watch out for the hidden salt in processed foods.

Foods high in sodium:

1. Frozen meals

2. Cured deli meats

3. Cheese

4. Sauces, condiments, salad dressings

5. Breads

6. Cereals

7. All sodas, especially diet soda

Want a "healthy" sandwich? White bread, cured meats, processed cheese, and mayo give you easily over 1,500 milligrams of sodium. One slice of pizza has over 700 milligrams of sodium.

The point here isn't to obsess, the point is to be aware that most times when you step on that scale and you've seen a weight gain it's more than likely the sodium you've had from eating out or having too much processed food. Eat real foods for real results and keep your sodium and potassium in check. And by real foods, whole foods, I'm talking about having food that is as close to its natural state as possible. Remember, if it has a short expiration date it is probably good for you and if its expiration date is a year from now, it's probably not.

7/11 Combo Buffer Zone

Profile 5

Name: Patricia Martin   **Height:** 5'2"

Profession: English Teacher   **Weight:** 164 lbs. (was 173)

Age: 54   **Ideal Weight:** 110 lbs.

Marital Status: Married   **Children:** 5

Living Arrangements: House   **Exercise:** Yes

Commute: 40 minutes

Patricia breezed through the 7/14 combo Buffer Zone and lost nine pounds her first thirty days. She's pumped! Her biggest sacrifice, if you want to call it that, was giving up her Dean's French Onion dip and Ruffles potato chip habit that she enjoyed while watching her favorite prime-time shows. Once she dropped her late-night snacking and she increased her workout routine from three to seven days a week, she's never had so much energy. Patricia has been averaging over fifteen hours a day on her Buffer Zones to easily surpass her 20 percent goal of 33.6 hours of fat fuel burning a week (remember: the first ten hours of a Buffer Zone are not counted in the fat fuel burning calculations; so fifteen hours minus ten hours transition to five hours of fat fuel and five hours a night times seven days in a week is thirty-five hours).

After the thirty-day transition period, Patricia has chosen the 7/11 combo Buffer Zone to take it to the next level. She wants to add another fifteen hours of fat fuel burning so she can be on the 70/30 plan (70 percent glycogen fuel, daily food intake and 30 percent triglycerides, fat fuel, adipose tissue/stored body fat). She's going to be skipping three suppers a week to get the extra hours.

Patricia's concerns:

1. Her husband is overweight and refusing to go on the Buffer Zone as well. Patricia's new healthy lifestyle is causing friction in their relationship, as her husband (who loves to cook) isn't doing anything to maintain his health. He is extremely overweight, doesn't exercise, and drinks way too much. In a study released recently, couples who both drank or both abstained from alcohol were in more stable relationships. In couples that chose opposite lifestyles, the couples had a higher divorce rate. Patricia has been doing her best to get her health back but it doesn't help when her husband walks in with a bucket of KFC (Kentucky Fried Chicken).

2. Some family vacations are coming up and Patricia is concerned how she will be able to stay on the Buffer Zone with all the traveling and exotic foods that will be available.

3. But Patricia's bigger concern has been maintaining her full-tank meals. She has eaten small meals for so long, it's hard for her to have over 50 percent of her caloric intake at one meal. The days she fails to eat enough on her full-tank

meals, she drags the rest of the day and gets more cravings at night. Her big fear is simple: can she get enough nutrition into her body if she starts skipping some suppers?

Solutions

One of the hardest things to do in the whole world is to watch somebody drowning in shallow water because they are too hard-headed to stand up for themselves. Patricia's main obstacle to getting her health back is, sadly, her husband. Marriage is a team sport and if he is mocking her diet and not helping, it makes it much more difficult on her. However, in this instance her actions will need to speak louder than her words. Once her husband sees that his wife is actually losing and keeping the weight off, he's more likely to join in.

As for the vacations, Patricia needs to stick to her Buffer Zone as best as she can. If she doesn't get enough Buffer Zone hours in one day, she can make them up the next. The main thing for her to remember is to not throw in the towel and declare vacations as time to cheat. She'll only be hurting herself. Even if while doing her best, she does gain a pound or two, it won't be a big deal in the big scheme of things.

As a mother, Patricia has learned to do without for her family and that has included being less satisfied. Patricia has been less of herself to make those around her "more" happy. Patricia has got to learn how to eat her meals slowly. She usually scarfs her food down so quickly just so she can begin the cleaning up process. She isn't truly honoring dinnertime. That requires allowing the body to have thirty minutes to one hour to leisurely enjoy her full-tank meal. If she does this, she will be able to get enough nutrition in and hit her caloric needs. Moms who are used to feeding a family can easily get stuck in serving mode and forget to pause and take care of their own needs. Believe it or not, one of the top reasons women fail to lose weight is because they aren't getting enough calories—not getting too many. Then they just end up getting sick and give up on their diet and themselves.

The Buffer Zone isn't an all-or-nothing diet. It's a diet where the frequency and timing of your meals are changed more so than the content. If Patricia cannot learn to slow down and finish her full-tank meals, she will have to go back to the 7/14 combo in order to get her daily requirement of nutrients. Our goal isn't just to lose weight, it's to be healthy. How we get to our ideal body weight is just as important as reaching it.

CHAPTER 13

Primers and Full-Tanks

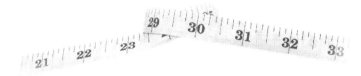

On the 7/14, 7/11, or 7/7 (coming up in chapter 14) the fuel your body runs on—its octane, if you will—comes in the form of primer meals, full-tank meals, and fat fuel. Primer meals are 20 to 40 percent of your daily caloric intake and full-tank meals are 60 to 80 percent (60 percent can go up to 80 percent when you're on the 7/7). If your meals are designed correctly, you'll be able to use your daily food allowance to keep you going when you are on the move and your fat fuel to keep you alive, when you're resting or on standby (sleeping). If you burn up your daily intake food too quickly, the Buffer Zones are going to leave you unsatisfied and unhealthy. As we discussed already, well-designed primers get you up to five hours of fuel (three hours to go, two hours of rest) and full-tank meals get you ten hours of fuel (eight hours of go time, two hours of rest).

That said, could you have all of your calories via a bag of M&Ms? No. Those M&Ms would burn brightly for about twenty minutes and then all the long-term energy would be gone. That's a quality you see in junk food or pure sugar—rush of energy, like a bright flash of light, then darkness. If we don't design slow-burning octane fuel for our bodies, we not only won't get the nutrients our bodies need but we will also feel exhausted and hungry. Bodies that are asked to run on only fossil fuel (fat fuel) run sluggish. So that begs the question: what exactly are the nutrients we need on a daily basis and which foods will help us get what we need to succeed?

Here's the simple list, known as the Six Essential Daily Nutrients.

1. Carbohydrates
2. Protein
3. Fat
4. Vitamins
5. Minerals
6. Water

We've already touched on this list before but we really haven't dug deep. Think about all the questions it would be helpful to know.

1. Which are the best carbohydrates for you and why?

2. Does it matter what time of the day you eat your carbs?

3. How should carbs be mixed with the other five essential nutrients?

4. What is the best way to get our protein?

5. What are the healthy fats and what is the best way to get them?

6. What are the vitamins I need and what is the best way to deliver them to my body?

7. What minerals does my body require and what is the best way to deliver them?

8. How much water should I drink a day? Does it matter how I portion the water I drink? Does it matter when I drink my water? Can I drink too much water? What is the best way to get my water? What is the deal with vitamin water?

9. What foods should I consume to get my Six Essential Daily Nutrients?

10. What happens if I become nutrient deficient? How would I know if I'm getting enough nutrients or too much?

I've said it before and I'll say it again, food is a drug. Too much, too little, or even at the wrong time, all can be harmful to us. So, let's roll up our sleeves and get into the chemistry of food. We'll start by answering the previous questions and then

looking at some sample classic breakfast and lunch primers and
well-designed, full-tank meals.

  1. *Which are the best carbohydrates for you and why?*

The first thing to understand is that a carbohydrate is a molecule
made up of carbon, hydrogen, and oxygen atoms. Within the
larger group of six essential nutrients, carbohydrates are part of
a subgroup of three macronutrients (protein and fat being the
other two). All carbohydrates fall into three categories:

Simple Sugars: These are very short-chain carbohydrates
found in the foods we eat. There is glucose that can be
easily found in sweets, cereals, or pasta. Lactose, which
is milk sugar; sucrose, which is table sugar; and fructose,
which is fruit sugar. Simple sugars are absorbed directly
into your blood stream during digestion.

Starches: These are long-chain glucose molecules. They, too,
will eventually be broken down to glucose as the main energy
source of the body. The advantage of starches over simple
sugars is that they are time delayed. Here's an example:
Starchy foods include potatoes, corn, peas, beans, whole
grains, and bananas. Because starches take longer for your
body to process, the fuel they provide keeps us going longer.

Fiber: While humans actually don't digest fiber, fiber
is critical to maintain a healthy and balanced digestive
system. There are two types of fiber we want in our diet;
soluble and insoluble. Soluble fiber dissolves with the
water in your digestive system and helps to regulate the

cholesterol in your blood. Besides dehydration, low fiber can lead to constipation, which is why slowly adding fiber to your diet can help keep you regular. Insoluble fiber doesn't break down in water and helps guide your food through your digestive system without any hiccups. Without insoluble fiber you wouldn't have healthy bowels.

Since fiber doesn't come from meat, fish, or any dairy products, you'll have to get all your fiber from plants. Soluble fiber is readily found in fruits and vegetables, especially bananas, apples, carrots, potatoes, and oats. Insoluble fiber comes from bran, cereals, and most nuts and seeds. The easiest way to keep the two different fibers straight in your head is to remember that soluble fiber slows digestion and helps you absorb all the nutrients you need from food and insoluble fiber puts more bulk "in" your stool so it passes through you more quickly.

When you think about what fiber does for us:

1. Helps us slow our digestive system so we can absorb all the nutrients we need to stay healthy

2. Transports all the nonessential waste through our bodies and out so we can keep our plumbing running smoothly

You'd think we'd all add more fiber to our diets. Sadly, we typically only get 15 to 18 milligrams of fiber daily when we should be aiming for 30 milligrams. The carbohydrates that are best for us are the ones high in fiber and low in sugar (simple sugars). The ones that are less healthy are the opposite: high in sugar and low in fiber. That's why an apple a day keeps the doctor away, but a glass of apple juice is drinking pure sugar. Good carbs? It's all in the fiber. P.S.: Soluble fiber additives that dissolve in water do little to help constipation. If we are looking to become regular again, you'll need insoluble fiber, not soluble.

2. Does it matter what time of the day you eat your carbs?

Yes and no. Carbs need to be consumed in a mix with the other macronutrients. Fifty-five percent carbs, 30 percent fats (no more than 7 percent saturated fats), and 15 percent protein.

There is no time that carbs should be eaten in isolation or they spike your insulin levels. In 2004, John Ivy, PhD, and Robert Portman, PhD, published a study entitled *Nutrient Timing* where they argued that having most or all your carbs earlier in the day reduced fat productions versus having heavy carb loading at night before you go to bed. Since then, enough studies have disproven some of their research and show that carbs taken at any time, as long as they are eaten with a well-balanced meal and within your personal caloric requirements are fine. Where their research does ring true is with carb snacking or late-night carb eating. If carbs are not balanced out with the other five essential nutrients (protein, fat, water, minerals, and vitamins) you will add body fat. No buffer zone in the world can help you if all you eat is 100 percent of your calories from carbs or from fat or protein. It always comes back to a proper balance.

3. How should carbs be mixed with other nutrients?

Simple sugars should be back loaded. Think of the order in which we typically order a meal; appetizer/salad, entrée, dessert. Since simple sugars are absorbed so quickly, it's always best to have them after your body is stabilized with complex carbs, fats, and protein. This prevents an insulin spike and jolt to your metabolism. Complex carbs can be eaten before or with other nutrients. It's just inadvisable to only eat complex or simple carbs in isolation. The reason we need protein and fat is because there are essential amino acids and fatty acids our bodies require to stay healthy. If we don't get them or some of them at every eating event, we run the risk of clogging our arteries with too much carbs. Of the twenty essential amino acids our bodies need, eight of them can only come from protein and there are two fatty acids, linoleic and alpha-linolenic, that cannot be synthesized by the human body. Think of water, H_2O: without the hydrogen or oxygen, all we got is gas. Blend your macronutrients and always have simple carbs after, not before, any meal and you'll be okay.

4. What is the best way to get our protein?

There are so many ways to get our protein: red meat, dairy products, energy bars, protein shakes, fish, poultry, beans, tofu, soy products, seeds, and nuts. If you've been on a western diet (high intake of red meat, refined sugars, and saturated fat with little or no fiber) getting enough protein isn't your problem; it's getting too much and not enough quality. Just like with carbs, not all protein is created equal.

Let's look at red meat. It's protein but also rich in saturated fat. Then there is the question of the type of red meat you eat. Industry-raised animals rarely have access to the outdoors and are juiced with growth hormones, antibiotics, genetically modified organisms (GMOs), and pesticides. Of course, one solution would be to eat organic, grass-fed red meat and dairy from animals that get to live in a more natural environment, but the best thing you can do is add variety. Red meat cannot be your only source of protein. Fish is super high in protein and low in saturated fat. Poultry is a winner if you remove the skin that has all the fat. Beans are great not only because they are loaded with protein, but also add fiber. And, of course, vegetarians can eat soy and tofu products.

According to the Dietary Reference Intake, the ideal amount of protein we should get a day is 0.8 grams of protein per kilogram or .36 grams per pound. For example, I weigh 178 pounds (178 × .36 = 64.08 grams). Recent studies show that the average person is eating twice the amount of protein they require. Men are eating over 100 grams a day. Women are a little better; they're eating approximately 70 grams. Fifteen percent of our diet should be protein, but it turns out we are having over 30 percent. This excess of protein is stressing out our bodies, adding weight, and trashing our kidneys. Besides variety, the most important thing you can do when it comes to protein is lower your intake.

Here's how much protein is in the typical food we eat. You'll see just how easy it is to go over.

- Red meat, pork, poultry, and seafood range between 6 to 9 grams of protein per ounce.

- Seeds and nuts contain 4 to 8 grams of protein for one-quarter of a cup.

- Cooked beans range between 7 to 8 grams per half cup.

- Cooked grains (like oatmeal) range 5 to 7 grams per cup.

- Eggs have approximately 6 grams of protein per egg.

- Most vegetables have about 2.5 grams per half cup.

One 9-ounce steak will put you over 70 grams of protein. A typical juicy hamburger has 20 grams; heck, even a pork chop has 24 grams. Think of the typical plate of food you eat; is 50 percent of it some type of protein? My guess is yes. That's got to be cut in half and we have to increase our variety so we don't get too much added saturated fat or excess sodium. One healthy 3-ounce serving of lean beef, pork, or poultry is about the size of a deck of playing cards. A good thing to remember before you dig into your meat meal.

5. What are healthy fats and what is the best way to get them?

Fats are either saturated or unsaturated. Saturated fats are unhealthy for you and will raise your low-density lipoprotein (LDL) cholesterol levels and lower your high-density lipoprotein (HDL). High levels of LDL cholesterol increase your risk of cardio-vascular disease. Good cholesterol (HDL) is in a counterbalance with bad cholesterol (LDL). When one goes up, the other goes down and vice versa. In order to keep our good (HDL) levels high (above 60 milligrams per deciliter [mg/dL]) we have to have three times more unsaturated fat in our diets versus saturated fat. A poor HDL level is below 40 mg/dL. Unsaturated fats come in two varieties:

- *Monounsaturated fatty acids:* Also referred to as (MUFAs) are good fats that are liquid at room temperature but turn solid when refrigerated. These are the fats that improve blood cholesterol levels, decrease heart disease, and help regulate insulin levels to control blood sugar spikes that can be harmful to you if you have type 2 diabetes. They can be found in olive oil, canola oil, and peanut oil.

- *Polyunsaturated fatty acids:* These are dietary fats that, like monounsaturated fats, are helpful for normal growth and development of your body. They can be found mostly in fish, leafy greens, seeds, and nuts. Like all fats, they are packed with energy, coming in at nine calories per gram—over twice the energy punch of carbs or protein that are four calories per gram. Maybe that's why fat tastes so good, because somewhere in our brain we know they are energy dynamos. Salmon, mackerel, herring, and trout are rich in polyunsaturated fats. We get our essential omega-6 and omega-3 fatty acids from polyunsaturated fats.

- *Saturated fats:* These are the bad guys. They have a higher melting point; they are solid at room temperature and raise our risk of cardiovascular disease. They raise the bad cholesterol (LDL) and lower the good cholesterol (HDL). The simple conclusion would be to just eat healthy fat and avoid bad saturated fat. Here's the problem: You can't have one without the other. They almost always travel together. The only thing you can do is try to pick the foods that have a higher percentage of monounsaturated and polyunsaturated fat than saturated fat. Let me give you an example: Cheese, whole milk, 2 percent milk, ice cream, and even light ice cream is over 60 percent saturated fat and under 40 percent unsaturated fat. Cheese pizza is bad for you as it comes in at 60 percent saturated fat, sausage pizza is less bad as it is 40 percent saturated fat, but an oatmeal cookie is only 22 percent saturated fat. Yellow birthday cake is 60 percent saturated fat and a pastry is 50 percent.

Take a look at the full list of saturated and unsaturated fats from Wikipedia:

Food	Saturated	Mono-unsaturated	Poly-unsaturated
	As weight percent (%) of total fat		
Cooking Oils			
Canola oil	8	64	40
Corn oil	13	24	59
Olive oil	7	78	15
Sunflower oil	11	20	69
Soybean oil	15	24	58
Peanut oil	17	46	32
Rice Bran oil	25	38	37
Coconut oil	87	13	1
Dairy Products			
Cheese, regular	64	29	3
Cheese, light	60	30	0
Milk, whole	62	28	4
Milk, 2%	62	30	0
Ice cream, gourmet	62	29	4
Ice cream, light	62	29	4
Meats			
Beef	33	38	5
Ground sirloin	38	44	4

Pork chop	35	44	8
Ham	35	49	16
Chicken breast	29	34	21
Chicken	34	23	30
Turkey breast	30	20	30
Turkey drumstick	32	22	30
Fish, orange roughy	23	15	46
Salmon	28	33	28
Hot dog, beef	42	48	5
Hot dog, turkey	28	40	22
Burger, fast food	36	44	6
Cheeseburger, fast food	43	40	7
Breaded chicken sandwich	20	39	32
Grilled chicken sandwich	26	42	20
Sausage, Polish	37	46	11
Sausage, turkey	28	40	22
Pizza, sausage	41	32	20
Pizza, cheese	60	28	5
Nuts			
Almonds, dry roasted	9	65	21
Cashews, dry roasted	20	59	17
Macadamia, dry roasted	15	79	2
Peanuts, dry roasted	14	50	31
Pecans, dry roasted	8	62	25
Flaxseeds, ground	8	23	65
Sesame seeds	14	38	44
Soybeans	14	22	57
Sunflower seeds	11	19	66
Walnuts, dry roasted	9	23	63

Sweets and Baked Goods			
Candy, chocolate bar	59	33	3
Candy, fruit chews	14	44	38
Cookie, oatmeal raisin	22	47	27
Cookie, chocolate chip	35	42	18
Cake, yellow	60	25	10
Pastry, Danish	50	31	14
Fats added during cooking or at the table			
Butter, stick	63	29	3
Butter, whipped	62	29	4
Margarine, stick	18	39	39
Margarine, tub	16	33	49
Margarine, light tub	19	46	33
Lard	39	45	11
Shortening	25	45	26
Chicken fat	30	45	21
Beef fat	41	43	3
Dressing, blue cheese	16	54	25
Dressing, light Italian	14	24	58
Other			
Egg yolk fat	36	44	16
Avocado	16	71	13

In every one of the above examples you'll see that you can't have a little good fat without a little bad and vice versa. The thing to remember is only 30 percent of your calories can come from fat and only 25 percent (approximately) of your dietary fat can be saturated. If you indulge in some cheese pizza today, you may want to just settle for some dry roasted almonds tomorrow to balance the scale.

Oh, and one more thing: trans fats. These are fats that are uncommon in nature but can be produced industrially from vegetable fats. Since the 1950s, trans fats have been showing up in baking foods, snack foods, and fast foods. As a rule, avoid them. If you can't, dilute them with enough good/real food to make sure you get the nutrients your body requires.

(*Note:* The FDA recommends eating eight to twelve ounces of fish a week to take the place of other protein but does recommend to check the mercury levels of the fish you're eating. Mercury is a naturally occurring element found in water, air, soil, fish, shellfish, and animals that eat fish. Fish and shellfish are the main sources of mercury exposure in humans. Mercury at high levels can be harmful to the brain, heart, kidneys, lungs, and immune system. Also, high levels of mercury can be harmful to the IQ of unborn babies. Fish low in mercury are salmon, tilapia, tuna (canned), cod, and catfish. Fish that are high in mercury are tilefish, shark, swordfish, and king mackerel. Fish that have less than ½ milligram of mercury per kilogram are safe for you to eat without worry. Fish that have ½ milligram to 1 milligram of mercury per kilogram should be consumed in moderation (6 to 8 ounces a week) and fish that are over 1 milligram of mercury per kilogram you shouldn't have more than 4 ounces a week.

Here's a list of some of the most popular seafood and their EPA maximum weekly recommended limits:

- Albacore (canned)—6 ounces or less

- Anchovies—6 ounces or less

- Bass (Chilean)—6 ounces or less

- Bluefish—6 ounces or less
- Butterfish—30 ounces or less
- Carp—14 ounces or less
- Catfish—40 ounces or less
- Clams—unlimited
- Cod (Atlantic)—20 ounces or less
- Crab—30 ounces or less
- Crawfish—20 ounces or less
- Croaker (Atlantic)—20 ounces or less
- Flounder/Sole—30 ounces or less
- Grouper—6 ounces or less
- Haddock (Atlantic)—60 ounces or less
- Halibut—8 ounces or less
- King Mackerel—3 ounces or less
- Lobster (in general)—16 ounces or less
- Lobster (Northern United States)—8 ounces or less
- Mackerel (Spanish Gulf)—4 ounces or less
- Mackerel (Spanish Atlantic)—12 ounces or less
- Mahi-mahi—12 ounces or less
- Marlin—4 ounces or less
- Monkfish—12 ounces or less
- Orange roughy—4 ounces or less
- Oysters—80 ounces or less

- Perch (fresh water)—16 ounces or less
- Pollack—20 ounces or less
- Salmon (canned)—unlimited
- Salmon (fresh or frozen)—150 ounces or less
- Sardines—120 ounces or less
- Scallops—40 ounces or less
- Shark—2 ounces or less
- Skate—16 ounces or less
- Snapper—12 ounces or less
- Squid—30 ounces or less
- Swordfish—2 ounces or less
- Tilapia—200 ounces or less
- Tilefish (Atlantic)—14 ounces or less
- Tilefish (Gulf of Mexico)—2 ounces or less
- Trout (Freshwater)—24 ounces or less
- Trout (Ocean)—8 ounces or less
- Tuna (Canned)—16 ounces or less
- Tuna (Canned Albacore)—6 ounces or less
- Tuna (Troll-caught)—6 ounces or less
- Tuna (Albacore)—6 ounces or less
- Tuna (In general)—6 ounces or less
- Tuna (Big Eye)—3 ounces or less
- Whitefish—30 ounces or less

All of the preceding calculations were based on a person weighing approximately 180 pounds. Obviously if you weigh ninety pounds, these numbers would be cut in half. If you weigh more, your capacity would also increase.

6. *What are the vitamins I need and what is the best way to deliver them to my body?*

A vitamin is a vital nutrient that we require in small amounts to keep us healthy. An organic chemical compound is called a vitamin when the organism (us) cannot synthesize the compound but must get it from our diet.

- **Vitamin A:** Must be taken with food since it is a fat-soluble vitamin. Fat-soluble vitamins won't break down and be absorbed in water/empty stomach. The recommended dietary allowance for vitamin A is nine hundred micrograms. The upper limit is three thousand micrograms. The best way to get vitamin A is liver, yellow fruits, squash, carrots, spinach, fish, milk, and leafy vegetables.

- **Vitamin B$_1$:** Is water soluble and can be taken without food. The recommended dietary allowance of vitamin B$_1$ is 1.2 mg (there is no recognized daily limit). The best way to get your vitamin B$_1$ is with pork, brown rice, oatmeal, vegetables, potatoes, eggs, and liver.

- **Vitamin B$_2$:** Is water soluble and can be taken without food. The recommended dietary allowance for vitamin B$_2$ is 1.3 milligrams (there is no recognized daily limit). The best way to get vitamin B$_2$ is through dairy products, bananas, popcorn, green beans, and asparagus.

- **Vitamin B$_3$:** Is water soluble and can be taken without food. The recommended dietary allowance for vitamin B$_3$ is sixteen milligrams. The upper limit is thirty-five milligrams. It is important to note that there are dire consequences to taking too much vitamin B$_3$. Permanent liver damage can occur if you take over two grams. Since there are one thousand milligrams in a gram, it would take fifty-seven times the daily limit to hurt yourself. While it may seem impossible to overdose on vitamin B$_3$ with your daily diet, many vitamin manufacturers create megadoses when they sell their product (overkill). For example, Nature Made sells niacin (B$_3$) in five-hundred-milligram tablets. If you took four pills, you would potentially damage your liver. It is always best to get your vitamins from food whenever possible. The best way to get vitamin B$_3$ is through fish, meat, eggs, many vegetables, mushrooms, and tree nuts.

- **Vitamin B$_5$:** Is water soluble and can be taken on an empty stomach. The recommended dietary allowance for vitamin B$_5$ is five milligrams (there is no recognized daily limit). The best way to get vitamin B$_5$ is with meat, broccoli, and avocados.

- **Vitamin B$_6$:** Is water soluble and can be taken without food. The recommended dietary allowance for vitamin B$_6$ is 1.3 to 1.7 milligrams. The upper limit is one hundred milligrams. The best way to get vitamin B$_6$ is with meat, vegetables, bananas, and tree nuts.

- **Vitamin B$_7$:** Is water soluble and can be taken without food. The recommended dietary allowance for vitamin B$_7$ is thirty micrograms. (Note: One thousand micrograms is one milligram and one thousand milligrams is one gram. So when we are talking about thirty micrograms, we are talking about a very small [yet essential] daily requirement.) There is no recognized daily limit for vitamin B$_7$. The best way to get vitamin B$_7$ is through raw egg yolk, liver, peanuts, and leafy green vegetables.

- **Vitamin B$_9$:** Is water soluble and can be taken without food. The recommended dietary allowance for vitamin B$_9$ is four hundred micrograms. The upper limit is one thousand micrograms. The best way to get vitamin B$_9$ is through leafy vegetables, pasta, bread, cereal, and liver.

- **Vitamin B$_{12}$:** Is water soluble and can be taken without food. The recommended dietary allowance for vitamin B$_{12}$ is 2.4 micrograms. There is no recognized daily limit. The best way to get vitamin B$_{12}$ is in meat, fish, poultry, eggs, and milk.

- **Vitamin C:** Is water soluble and can be taken without food. The recommended dietary allowance for vitamin C is ninety milligrams. The upper limit is two thousand milligrams. The best way to get vitamin C is many different fruits, vegetables, and liver.

- **Vitamin D:** Must be taken with food since it is a fat-soluble vitamin. The recommended dietary allowance for vitamin D is ten micrograms. The upper limit is fifty micrograms. One of the things I noticed is that the vitamin D supplements that are out there are labeled in International Units. So, if our daily allowance is ten micrograms that would equal four hundred International Units (IU). The upper limit would be two thousand IU. In order to have a serious health risk and overdose on vitamin D, you'd have to take over ten thousand IUs a day for over three months or over three hundred thousand IUs in a twenty-four-hour period. The best way to get your vitamin D is with fifteen minutes a day of daylight. Don't forget sunscreen! Sunscreen doesn't affect vitamin D production. Besides sunlight, vitamin D can be obtained through fortified milk, fish, eggs, liver, and mushrooms.

- **Vitamin E:** Must be taken with food since it is a fat-soluble vitamin. The recommended daily allowance for vitamin E is fifteen milligrams. The upper limit is one thousand milligrams. The best way to get vitamin E is through many fruits, vegetables, nuts, and seeds.

- **Vitamin K:** Must be taken with food since it is a fat-soluble vitamin. The recommended dietary allowance for vitamin K is 120 micrograms and there is no recognized daily limit. If you weigh more, your capacity would also increase. Vitamin K is found in leafy green vegetables.

7. *What minerals does my body require and what is the best way to deliver those minerals?*

- **Calcium:** We need calcium to build strong bones and teeth. On top of that, calcium plays a vital part in nerve transmissions and muscle functions. Without calcium, our hearts couldn't signal and time the proper contractions. When it comes to our hearts, having calcium is a matter of life and death. Even our digestive system can't run properly without calcium. As a general rule, mineral supplements should be taken on an empty stomach. That way the acids in your stomach can break them up so they can quickly be absorbed. There are a few exceptions and of course we will mention those here. The recommended dietary allowance for calcium is one thousand milligrams. The upper limit is 2,500 milligrams. The best way to get your calcium is through dairy products, eggs, canned fish with bones (salmon, sardines), nuts, seeds, tofu, thyme, oregano, dill, cinnamon, and leafy green vegetables.

- **Potassium:** As we talked about before, potassium is the counterbalance to sodium. It is an essential electrolyte that coregulates adenosine triphosphate (ATP), the molecular unit of currency of intracellular energy transfer. Without potassium and sodium working together we wouldn't be able to transport chemical energy within cells for metabolism. The recommended dietary allowance for potassium is 4,700 milligrams and there is no recognized daily limit. The best way to get potassium is through sweet potatoes, tomatoes, beans, lentils, dairy products, seafood, bananas, prunes, carrots, and oranges.

- **Sodium:** A vital systemic electrolyte that is essential in co-regulating ATP with potassium. While our bodies need five hundred milligrams, we shouldn't exceed 2,300 milligrams. The main source for most people in getting sodium is table salt. In general, our problem isn't a lack of sodium but too much. In merely one large glass of whole milk (two cups) you'll find half the sodium your body requires. The average American consumes 4,500 milligrams of sodium a day, twice the maximum value.

• **Magnesium:** There are over three hundred biochemical reactions that your body needs magnesium for. Like calcium, our bodies use magnesium to support muscle and nerve function, as well as to keep your heart beating and bones strong. The recommended dietary allowance of magnesium for women is between 310 to 360 milligrams a day and for men it is 400 milligrams. What's interesting is it's safe to get too much magnesium from our food but it's dangerous when it is taken in the form of a supplement. The highest upper limit for a magnesium supplement is 350 milligrams for adults. The best way to get our magnesium is through green leafy vegetables (like spinach), nuts, beans, peas, soybeans, whole grain cereals, peanut butter, and avocados.

Trace Minerals

Iron, zinc, magnesium, copper, iodine, chromium, molybdenum, selenium, and cobalt are trace elements that our body requires. In the following chart, I list the recommended dietary allowance, upper limits, and best source.

Dietary Element	Recommended	Upper Limits	Best Source
Iron	18 mg	45 mg	Meat, seafood, nuts, dark chocolate, beans
Zinc	15 mg	40 mg	Oysters, red meat, poultry, nuts, whole grains, dairy products
Manganese	2 mg	350 mg	Grains, legumes, leafy vegetables, seeds, nuts, tea, coffee
Copper	2 mg	11 mg	Seafood, oysters, liver, nuts, seeds, some whole grains, legumes
Iodine	0.15 mg	1.1 mg	Grains, eggs, seaweed (kelp or kombu), iodized salt
Chromium	.12 mg	N/A	Broccoli, grape juice, meat, whole grain products
Selenium	0.07 mg	0.4 mg	Brazil nuts, seafood, organ meats, meats, grains, dairy products, eggs
Cobalt	None	N/A	Found in vitamin B_{12}

8. *How much water should I drink a day? Does it matter how I portion the water I drink? Does it matter when I drink water? Can I drink too much water? What is the best way to get my water? What is the deal with vitamin water?*

Everyone has their own unique chemistry so there is no way to say exactly how much water you should drink. That said, I'm not sure anyone has died by drinking eight cups (eight ounces) of water spread throughout the day. I recommend downing sixteen ounces of water after you wake up and have weighed in. Since it takes a full hour for water to go from your gut to your muscles, it's always great to hydrate before a workout. Our kidneys can eliminate about a liter (33.81 ounces) of fluid an hour. So it's wise to not try to get all your fluids in at once. Too much water will dilute the sodium and nutrients in your blood and it can be fatal. There are reported cases of people dying after downing six liters of water over a three-hour time period. There is a saying: "Dose makes the poison." While it isn't completely correct because there are things in this world like lead or arsenic that are poisonous at any dose, but it is true of water. Six liters consumed all at once kills 50 percent of the people that attempt it.

Of course, the opposite of overhydration is dehydration. Dehydration occurs when you lose more fluid than you take in. Typically, dehydration occurs when you are in a hot climate and symptoms include vomiting, diarrhea, excessive sweating, and fever. But the reality is anyone can get dehydrated if they just forget to drink enough fluids throughout the day. The best times to get your water are when you wake up; with your front-loaded meals; before a workout; after a workout; when you're thirsty; feeling ill or tired; and three to four hours before bedtime. One of water's main functions is removing waste from our system, so it's a good idea to give your body a chance to clean itself out before you call it a day.

Vitamin water, soup, soda, or any type of liquid does count toward maintaining hydration levels. That even includes eating watermelon. Just keep an eye on caloric intake events. On the Buffer Zone, we only have a max of one front-loaded, full-tank meal and two primer meals to get our calories. Sipping on any drinks with added sugar will disrupt the Buffer Zone if they aren't tied with one of our meals. Coffee (with just a dash of milk) or non-sweetened ice tea is okay.

9. *What foods should I consume to get my Six Essential Daily Nutrients?*

There are six food groups that should all be a part of our daily food intake if we are going to get our essential daily nutrients. They are:

1. Fruits

2. Vegetables

3. Grains

4. Dairy

5. Protein

6. Oils

If we use two thousand calories as a daily caloric intake average, then that would mean we need two cups of fruits, two and one-half cups of vegetables, six ounces of grains, three cups of dairy, five and one-half ounces of protein, and six teaspoons of oils a day.

Let's go over some examples as what counts as an ounce, a cup, or a teaspoon of our main food groups. The following examples and tips are provided by the u.s. Department of Agriculture (usda).

Fruits

Food	Common portions and 1 cup equivalents
Apple	½ large (3¼" diameter)
	1 small (2¼" diameter)
	1 cup sliced or chopped, raw or cooked
Applesauce	1 cup
Banana	1 cup sliced
	1 large (8" or 9" long)
Cantaloupe	1 cup diced or melon balls
Grapes	1 cup, whole or cut up
	32 seedless grapes
Grapefruit	1 medium (4" diameter)
	1 cup of sections
Mixed fruit	1 cup diced or sliced, raw or canned, drained
Orange	1 large (3¹⁄₁₆" diameter)
	1 cup of sections
Orange (Mandarin)	1 cup canned, drained
Peach	1 large (2¾" diameter)
	1 cup sliced or diced, raw, cooked, or canned, drained
Pineapple	1 cup, chunks, sliced, crushed, raw, cooked, or canned, drained
Plum	1 cup sliced, raw or cooked
	3 medium or 2 large plums
Strawberries	About 8 large berries
	1 cup, whole, halved, or sliced, fresh or frozen
Watermelon	1 small (1" thick)
	1 cup, diced, or balls

Food	Common portions and 1 cup equivalents
Dried fruit (raisins, prunes, apricots, etc.)	½ cup dried fruit
100% fruit juice (orange, apple, grape, grapefruit, etc.)	1 cup

Tips for consuming fruits

- Select fresh, frozen, canned, and dried fruit more often than juice. If you do choose juice, make sure it's 100 percent fruit juice and not a blend.

- Enjoy a wide variety of fruits and maximize taste and freshness by adapting your choices to what's in season.

- Use fruits in your salads and desserts.

Vegetables

Food	Common portions and 1 cup equivalents
Broccoli	1 cup chopped or florets 3 spears 5" long, raw or cooked
Greens (collards, mustard greens, turnip greens, kale)	1 cup cooked
Spinach	1 cup cooked 2 cups raw
Raw leafy greens (spinach, romaine, watercress, dark green leafy lettuce, endive, escarole)	2 cups raw

Food	Common portions and 1 cup equivalents
Carrots	1 cup, strips, sliced, or chopped, raw or cooked
	2 medium
	1 cup baby carrots (about 12)
Pumpkin	1 cup mashed, cooked
Red Peppers	1 cup, chopped, raw or cooked
	1 large pepper (3" diameter, 3¾" long)
Tomatoes	1 large raw whole (3")
	1 cup, chopped or sliced, raw, canned or cooked
Tomato Juice	1 cup
Sweet Potato	1 large baked (2¼" or more in diameter)
	1 cup, sliced or mashed, cooked
Winter squash (acorn, butternut, hubbard)	1 cup cubed, cooked
Dry beans and peas (like black beans, garbanzo, kidney, pinto, or soybeans or black-eyed and split peas)	1 cup, whole or mashed, cooked
Corn (yellow or white)	1 cup
	1 large ear (8" to 9" long)
Green peas	1 cup
White potatoes	1 cup, diced, mashed
	1 medium boiled or baked potato (2½" to 3" diameter)
Bean sprouts	1 cup cooked
Cabbage, green	1 cup, chopped or shredded, raw or cooked
Cauliflower	1 cup, pieces or florets, raw or cooked

Food	Common portions and 1 cup equivalents
Celery	1 cup, diced or sliced, raw or cooked 2 large stalks (11" to 12" long)
Cucumbers	1 cup, raw, sliced or chopped
Green or wax beans	1 cup cooked
Green peppers	1 cup, chopped, raw or cooked 1 large pepper (3" diameter, 3¾" long)
Lettuce, iceberg or head	2 cups, raw, shredded or chopped
Mushrooms	1 cup, raw or cooked
Onions	1 cup, chopped, raw or cooked
Summer squash or zucchini	1 cup cooked, sliced, or diced

Tips for Consuming Vegetables

- Include vegetables in all meals. Fresh, frozen, and canned vegetables all count.

- Add dark green, red, and orange vegetables to main and side dishes. Use dark and leafy greens to make salads.

- Beans and peas are a great source of fiber. Add beans or peas to salads, soups, and side dishes or serve as a main dish.

Grains

Food	1 ounce equivalent of grains	Common portions and ounce equivalents
Bagels	1" mini bagel	1 large bagel = 4 ounces
Biscuits	1 small (2" diameter)	1 large (3" diameter) = 2 ounces

Food	1 ounce equivalent of grains	Common portions and ounce equivalents
Breads	1 regular slice 1 small slice French 4 snack slices rye	2 regular slices = 2 ounces
Bulgar	½ cup, cooked	
Cornbread	1 small piece (2½" × 1¼" × 1¼")	1 medium piece (2½" × 2½" × 1¼") = 2 ounces
Crackers	5 whole wheat crackers, 2 rye crispbreads, 7 square or round crackers	
English muffins	½ muffin	1 muffin = 2 ounces
Oatmeal	½ cup cooked 1 packet instant	Trader Joe's steel cut oatmeal is 1 cup and counts as 2 ounces
Pancakes	1 pancake (4½" diameter) 2 small pancakes (3" diameter)	3 pancakes (4½" diameter) is 3 ounces
Popcorn	3 cups, popped	1 mini microwave bag or 100 calorie bag, popped = 2 ounces
Ready to eat breakfast cereal	1 cup flakes or rounds 1¼ cup, puffed	
Rice, pasta, spaghetti, macaroni noodles	½ cup cooked, 1 ounce dry	1 cup cooked = 2 ounces
Tortillas	1 small flour (6" diameter) 1 corn tortilla (6" diameter)	1 large tortilla (12" diameter) = 4 ounces

Tips for Consuming Grains

- Make sure at least half of all the grains you eat are whole grains.

- Substitute whole grain choices for refined grains in breakfast cereals, breads, crackers, rice, and pasta.

- Check product labels; is a grain with "whole" before its name listed first on the ingredients list?

Dairy

Food	1 cup equivalent of dairy	Common portions and cup equivalents
Milk	1 cup milk ½ cup evaporated milk	
Yogurt	1 regular container (8 fluid ounces) 1 cup yogurt	1 small container (6 ounces) is ¾ cup
Cheese	1½ ounces hard cheese (cheddar, mozzarella, Swiss, parmesan) ⅓ cup shredded cheese 2 ounces processed cheese (American) ½ cup ricotta cheese 2 cups cottage cheese	1 slice hard cheese is equal to ½ cup milk 1 slice processed cheese is equal to ⅓ cup milk ½ cup of cottage cheese is equal to ¼ cup milk
Milk-based desserts	1 cup pudding made with milk 1 cup frozen yogurt 1½ cups ice cream	1 scoop of ice cream is equal to ⅓ cup milk
Soy milk (soy beverage)	1 cup calcium-fortified soy milk	

Tips for Consuming Dairy

- Drink fat-free (skim) or low-fat (1%) milk.

- Choose fat-free or low-fat milk or yogurt more often than cheese.

- When selecting cheese, choose low-fat or reduced-fat version.

Protein

Food	1 ounce equivalent of protein	Common portions and ounce equivalents
Meats	1 ounce cooked lean beef 1 ounce cooked lean pork or ham	1 small steak (eye of round, filet) = 3½–4 ounces 1 small lean hamburger = 2–3 ounces
Poultry	1 ounce cooked chicken or turkey without skin 1 sandwich slice of turkey (4½" × 2½" × ⅛")	1 small chicken breast = 3 ounces ½ Cornish game hen = 4 ounces
Seafood	1 ounce cooked fish or shellfish	1 can of tuna, drained = 3–4 ounces 1 salmon steak = 4–6 ounces 1 small trout = 3 ounces
Eggs	1 egg	3 egg whites = 2 ounces 3 egg yolks = 1 ounce
Nuts and Seeds	½ ounce of nuts (12 almonds, 24 pistachios, 7 walnut halves) ½ ounce of seeds (pumpkin, sunflower, or squash seeds, hulled and roasted) 1 tablespoon peanut butter or almond butter	1 ounce of nuts or seeds = 2 ounces

Beans and peas	¼ cup cooked beans (black, kidney, pinto, or white beans) ¼ cup of cooked peas (chickpeas, cowpeas, lentils, or split peas) ¼ cup baked beans, refried beans ¼ cup (about 2 ounces) of tofu 2 tablespoons hummus	1 cup split pea soup = 2 ounces 1 cup lentil soup = 2 ounces 1 cup bean soup = 2 ounces 1 soy or bean burger patty = 2 ounces

Tips for Consuming Protein

- Eat a variety of food from the protein group.

- Eat seafood in place of meat or poultry twice a week.

- Select lean meat and poultry. Trim or drain fat from meat and remove poultry skin.

Oils

Oils	Amount of Food	Amount of Oil
Vegetable oils (canola, corn, cottonseed, olive, peanut, safflower, soybean, and sunflower)	1 tbsp.	3 tsp.
Foods Rich in Oils	**Amount of Food**	**Amount of Oil**
Margarine, soft (trans fat free)	1 tbsp.	2½ tsp.
Mayonnaise	1 tbsp.	2½ tsp.
Mayonnaise-type salad dressing	1 tbsp.	1 tsp.
Italian dressing	2 tbsp.	2 tsp.
Thousand Island dressing	2 tbsp.	2½ tsp.

Olives, ripe, canned	4 large	½ tsp.
Avocado	½ medium	3 tsp.
Peanut butter	2 tbsp.	4 tsp.
Peanuts, dry roasted	1 oz.	3 tsp.
Mixed nuts, dry roasted	1 oz.	3 tsp.
Cashews & almonds, dry roasted	1 oz.	3 tsp.
Hazelnuts	1 oz.	4 tsp.
Sunflower seeds	1 oz.	3 tsp.

Tips for Consuming Oils

- Choose soft margarines with zero trans fats made from liquid vegetable oil, rather than stick margarine or butter.

- Use vegetable oils (olive, canola, corn, soybean, peanut, safflower, sunflower) rather than solid fats (butter, shortening).

- Rather than just adding oil to the diet, replace solid fats with oils. Oils are a concentrated source of calories, so use oils in small amounts.

10. *What happens if I become nutrient deficient? How would I know if I'm getting enough nutrients or too much?*

Your body is always talking to you but sometimes we miss out on its subtle cues. Did you know that cracks on the corner of your mouth can be signs that you're not getting enough iron, zinc, and B-12 in your diet? (Eggs, salmon, and oysters are a good, quick fix.) Or did you know that hair loss or rashes indicate that you're not getting enough B-7? (Eggs will help you out here yet again). There are so many ways our bodies try telling us they are not happy. For example: red or white acne-like bumps on our arms, thighs, behind, and face can be telling us that we aren't getting our essential fatty acids, vitamin A, or vitamin D. Muscle cramps can be a sign of not enough magnesium, calcium, and potassium. (Eat some almonds or hazelnuts.) Here is a list of common telltale signs that our bodies aren't getting a balanced diet:

Signs You Need Additional Iron:
- Always feeling cold
- Lightheadedness
- Headaches
- Dizziness
- Pale skin
- Trouble breathing

Signs You Need Additional Calcium:
- Constant fatigue
- Muscle cramps
- Prolonged abdominal appetite (not hungry or always hungry)
- Development of osteoporosis (over a long period of time)

Sign You Need Additional Vitamin D:

- There are no absolute, clear symptoms that you're not getting enough vitamin D, with the exception of a lowered immune system that makes you more susceptible to getting colds and the flu

Signs You Need Additional Vitamin C:

- Depression
- Nosebleeds
- Bleeding gums
- High blood pressure
- Bruising easily
- Gingivitis

Signs You Need Additional Protein:

- Thinning hair or hair falling out
- Aching muscles
- Constantly sick
- Muscle loss

Signs You Need Additional Fiber:

- Constant hunger
- Constipation

Signs You Need Additional Vitamin A:

- Dry eyes
- Night blindness
- Dry, scaling skin
- Diarrhea

I'll say it again: as long as you strive to have approximately two and one-half cups of vegetables, two cups of fruits, six ounces of grains, three cups of dairy, five and one-half ounces of protein, and six teaspoons of oils a day, you have a healthy, balanced diet. That works out to be 55 percent carbs, 30 percent fats, and 15 percent protein over your one to two primer meals and one full-tank meal a day. Do that and you'll be giving your body the high-octane fuel it needs to go strong all day long.

CHAPTER 14

Buffer Zone 3
(Maximum Fat Burning)

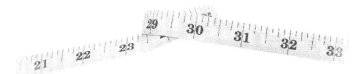

In Buffer Zone 1, we learned how to cut snacks from our lives and pack more nutrients in one full-tank meal (60 percent of our daily caloric intake) and two primer meals (20 percent each of our daily caloric intake). We learned that we were eating too frequently and at the wrong times. Buffer Zone 1 was about breaking longstanding habits and recalibrating our minds, bodies, and souls into a new, healthy lifestyle. We learned how to divvy up the week into an 80/20 plan; 80 percent of our weekly hours we learned to survive on just-in food (daily meals) and 20 percent of our time we learned to rely on old, stored fat fuel that we have in our bodies. Buffer Zone 1, the 7/14 (seven full-tank meals and fourteen primer meals) plan was the tool we used to turn our lives around.

After thirty days, we took it up a notch to Buffer Zone 2, 7/11. We dropped three primer dinners and added more fat burning time. The 7/11 Buffer Zone (Buffer Zone 2) accelerated our fat burning by 50 percent! We went from 20 percent fat burning time a week to 30 percent! At this point in the book, if you have successfully completed Buffer Zone 1 (thirty days) and a minimum of thirty days on Buffer Zone 2, you may be ready for the ultimate fat-burning challenge: Buffer Zone 3, the 7/7 Buffer Zone. This is where we drop all unnecessary primer dinners and switch to a stringent primer breakfast and dinner-for-lunch plan. The 7/7 Buffer Zone burns twice as much fat as Buffer Zone 1 and 33 percent more fat than Buffer Zone 2. It is not for the faint of heart. Many clients have never ever switched to Buffer Zone 2 or 3 and have had great success with reaching their weight-loss goals.

When I originally started on the Buffer Zone, I stayed on the 7/14 for quite a while before I ventured out. Many people will keep Buffer Zone 3 as their silver bullet to knock off their last tough five to ten pounds of body fat. My recommendation is to not switch Buffer Zones until you've hit a thirty-day plateau—that's thirty days in a row where your body resists losing any more weight.

For example, start with Buffer Zone 1 until you hit your first, full, thirty-day plateau, then switch to Buffer Zone 2 and stick with it until the next thirty-day plateau. Then when that happens, bring in the big guns of Buffer Zone 3 to break up the last, tough, hard-to-lose fat. The earliest I would switch Buffer

Zones is in one-month intervals; the first thirty days on Buffer Zone 1, then after thirty days Buffer Zone 2, and then Buffer Zone 3 after sixty days. Then you ride Buffer Zone 3 out until you hit your weight goal.

Buffer Zone 3, the 7/7 Buffer Zone, uses 40 percent of your stored fat to run your body a week. It is the quickest way to burn the most fat on your body safely. Once your body gets accustomed to running 60 percent on just-in fuel and 40 percent on fat fuel, your body becomes even more in tune. The nice thing about bodies is they can pretty much adapt to any environment or new habit in twenty-one to twenty-eight days (that's why I ask you to always give thirty days between Buffer Zones).

With the Buffer Zone, people all over the world will get their lives back and more time to follow their dreams. Life starts outside your comfort zone, and learning to let go of our high-frequency comfort eating habits is where our lives begin again. Let's take a look at Buffer Zone 3, the 7/7 Buffer Zone, in action!

$$* \quad * \quad *$$

When the subject of obesity (BMI 30+) in black Americans' lives comes up, it strikes a powerful chord. Everyone has an opinion on why the obesity rate among this segment of our population is so high. According to stateofobesity.org, African American adults are 1.5 times as likely to be obese compared with white adults. Approximately 47.8 percent of African Americans are obese (including 37.1 percent of men and 56.6 percent of women) compared with 32.6 percent of whites (including 32.4 percent of men and 32.8 percent of women).

More than 75 percent of African Americans are overweight (BMI 25+) or obese (including 66 percent of men and 82 percent of women) compared with 67.2 percent of Whites (including 71.4 percent of men and 63.2 percent of women).

If you are an African American woman living in the United States, there is only an 18 percent chance that you are at a healthy weight. Through my interviews, I blended commonalities to assemble the following voice. It would be impossible for me to tell everyone's story, but that didn't stop me from creating one voice to tell this story. I hope it resonates.

Typical 7/7 Buffer Zone Plan

Profile 6:

Name: Jazmin Jensen	**Height:** 5'7"
Profession: Comedian	**Weight:** 225 lbs.
Age: 36	**Ideal Weight:** Healthy Curvy
Marital Status: Separated	**Children:** 2
Living Arrangements: Brownstone	**Exercise:** Yes
Commute: Travels the country	

Hello, my name is Jazmin. I've been overweight since, well, since as long as I can remember. When I was young I was always complimented on my voracious appetite. I could really put away the food. I could keep up with both my big brothers. In school, I was teased because of my size. Schoolmates would make snorting sounds when they saw me. It hurt. But, I never let them know it. I'd make a joke of it. Daddy always told me that people could laugh at you or with you; I always tried to make sure it was with me. If I laughed too and squealed; it felt like we laughed together.

Laura was the girl in school all the boys seemed to pay attention to. She was skinny with long blonde hair. I called her Twiggy and told her when she grew up, nobody would want a body with no meat on it, so don't be jealous of me! In truth, I was jealous of her—at least until I started to fill out and I got my curves. Then the boys started paying attention to me.

It's funny but I've always had a complicated relationship with fat. At times, I'd feel so lonely and guilty as I finished off another bag of Cheetos and licked away the crumbs from my orange-stained fingers. At other times, I'd bump Laura with my hips when we walked down the halls and she'd crash into the lockers. With fat, I was weak and powerful at the same time. I stopped focusing on the weak part and embraced the powerful part.

Once I accepted the fact that I was genetically predisposed to be a big, beautiful, black woman, it took such a load off. I stopped counting calories, ate and drank whatever I wanted, and life was, well, heaven. Besides having curves that have curves, I'm sharp as a knife. My intellect got me into Columbia where I got my undergraduate and master's degrees in communications. I was big, beautiful, and smart. I had the answers and the wit to deal with everyone. When I left school, I decided to be a comedian, heck why not? I'd do what I do best: make fun of myself. I had a master's degree in doing that. And you know what, it paid well, too. When I was headlining in Vegas I felt a numbing in my left arm. I thought it must have fallen asleep, so I shook it.

It felt like an elephant was stepping on my chest and then, well, and then everything went black. Pun intended.

When I woke up I heard the sounds of a heart monitor and the rushing around of nurses and doctors helping patients. I was in some hospital and my brother, mommy, and daddy were by my side. So was a scrumptious-looking tall, dark, and handsome man who was looking at my chart.

"I'm Dr. Stevens. The blood supply to your heart was restricted and that's why you lost consciousness. The arteries to your heart have become thicker and harder due to plaque buildup," he said.

"You telling me I had a heart attack?" I asked.

"Well, yes, in layman's terms, that's exactly what you had." Dr. Stevens continued, "There appears to be no permanent damage to your heart muscle, but due to the elevated hypertension and skyrocketing LDL cholesterol, this could very well happen again, and next time you might not be so lucky . . ." Blah, blah, blah. He kept talking but I wasn't listening.

This man was probably just a hater; he probably had never seen a real woman before. Probably dates a skinny girl. Then I did hear something he said. "Are you listening to me? Am I getting through to you? You have high blood pressure; you also have Type II Diabetes. If you don't make major life changes right now, you're going to die."

At that moment, I saw my cousin come to the door with my kids; they had been crying. I heard my youngest ask if I was going to be okay. Here I was, surrounded by the people I love and it was food that put me here. I knew I needed to make changes but I grew up on fat-laden fast food. Grits, fried chicken, pecan pie, potato salad, corn chips, pizza, and hamburgers had been my friends. Salt and fat added flavor and curves. Did I really want to give those up? I hate vegetables. Some fruits are okay but there were more Pop Tarts and Oreos in our house than fresh fruit. Fruit was expensive. My folks didn't have money for that and then you had to eat it right away or it would go bad. Processed food was way more affordable and didn't spoil. How could food with such a long shelf life shorten mine? That's when it hit me: I am not my fat. Fat is killing me and I need to make a change for myself. My whole standup routine of self-hatred and making fun of myself had to stop. I couldn't justify hurting myself anymore. I had to change.

How Do We Help the Jazmins of This World?

Jazmin's story, to some degree, is a compilation of all of us. Early eating habits can definitely be driven by financial concerns. Our old-time food "favorites" were driven more by what was being offered at our dinner tables than necessarily having a sweet tooth. The lure of processed foods is that they are cheap and plentiful. A Happy Meal from McDonald's with a hamburger is $2.49. Two pounds of apples, two pounds of oranges, one pound of bananas, two pounds of potatoes, one pound of broccoli, one pound of cabbage, one pound of carrots, and one pound of romaine lettuce will run you an average of $13.38. By the time you add protein, grains, dairy, and oils (the four missing food groups) our grocery purchase will run way north of $20.00 to feed a family of four. If money is tight, people will opt for quick and easy.

When you eat a greasy burger or polish off a few glazed donuts, you don't see the damage you're doing to your body.

Non-nutritious processed food is a slow and silent killer. Within ninety minutes of giving your body fake food, your hunger comes raging back like a sleeping giant that was suddenly awakened, screaming and demanding for something nutritious. Then, you know what we do? We feed it more junk, more non-nutritious, fake, processed food. It's an endless cycle, one that ends with us becoming grazers, snackers, and nibblers. People that learn to never pass up an opportunity to eat and don't learn to say no to food. And when you never say no to something or someone, they become a spoiled brat. Instead of having mature, responsible appetites, we allow hunger to run the show. Anytime it starts to scream, we feed it to shut it up. Hunger is not our master.

The one thing the Jazmin in all of us has in common is a lack of satisfaction, not just with food, but life in general. When we feel disappointed (which is normal) do we eat right, time our meals correctly, and get a little physical exercise? Nope. We lay down, stop moving, and grab a bag of chips and salsa. We do what is cheap and easy. The Buffer Zone, be it the 7/14, 7/11, or 7/7, is expensive in terms of the commitment it takes and is hard. It takes self-discipline, something many of us lack.

While Jazmin is a fictionalized character, she does represent real people that have tougher hurdles than people who just eat too much healthy food. Too much of anything, even nutritious food, isn't good for you. For people that have been eating the wrong food their whole lives, the Buffer Zone (less meals timed effectively) won't work. The minute you go from being a person that grazes on food all day to a person eating one full-tank and one or two primer meals a day, you have less time and space to get the nutrition your body requires on a daily basis. So, if all you're eating for your meals is M&Ms, it won't be long before you wake Hunger, the sleeping giant. When our bodies get the nutrition they require, we learn to tame hunger. Hunger ends up working for us instead of against us.

True hunger builds very slowly. Instant hunger is emotional hunger. So, what does someone like Jazmin do? She learns to eat food that she has told herself her entire life she doesn't like. She has to get reacquainted with the fruits and vegetables she was deprived of as a child. After she has what is good for her and will give her long-term fuel, she can add the junk if she wants. The funny thing is, it won't take long for her body to send her a new message "I LOVE HIGH-OCTANE (nutritious) FOOD!" Pretty soon, she will lose a lot of the taste for the junk.

Jazmin's New Meal Plan 7/7

Jazmin gets two meals a day with Buffer Zone 3, the 7/7 Buffer Zone. A primer breakfast and a dinner for lunch. In those two meals, she has to satisfy all six food groups (fruits, vegetables, grains, dairy, protein, and oils) with a 55 percent distribution of carbs, 30 percent total fats (7 percent saturated, 23 percent unsaturated), and 15 percent protein. Two meals? That is a tall order. Let me break it down for you. That's two and one-half cups of vegetables, two cups of fruit, six ounces of grains, three cups of dairy, five and one-half ounces of protein, and six teaspoons of oils (two tablespoons). If Jazmin is going to pull this off, she's going to have to plan. Let's look at her schedule.

Breakfast

Normally a primer breakfast is 20 percent of our daily caloric intake, but with only two meals, we will have to bump that up to 30 to 40 percent. So many women have light breakfasts that they then have an impossible time getting all the rest of their calories with one full-tank meal at lunch. On the 7/7 Buffer Zone, each meal has got to be really thought out.

Let's look at a list of the food we don't want to see on our breakfast tables.

- Pancakes
- Sweet cereals
- White bread
- Biscuits
- Pastries/Donuts
- Fruit juices with preservatives
- Creamy or cheesy egg dishes like Eggs Benedict
- Cold cuts
- French toast
- Fried chicken/fried anything

SIMPLE RULE FOR BREAKFAST

Breakfast is for fresh. Make everything that you eat as fresh as possible. Fresh fruit, whole grains, poached, or boiled eggs. It's easy to fry an egg in oil but then there is way too much cholesterol. Google "healthy breakfasts" and you'll get a myriad of delicious options.

On the 7/7 Buffer Zone, lunch is far and away the biggest meal of the day and the last. Make it count. Do that by first timing it right. A solid breakfast will give you five hours of energy before falling off. A full-tank dinner for lunch will get you eight hours of go time and two hours of rest time (laying around and relaxing). If you have your full-tank meal too soon, you'll start hearing hunger raise its voice way before it's bedtime. If you go to bed at 10:00 p.m., then a noon full-tank meal is perfect. But if you tend to stay up late and see all of the *Tonight Show*, it could be way past eleven thirty before you doze off. If that's the case, having lunch at one thirty would suit you best. Real hunger, not emotional hunger, starts growling at ten hours after your last meal of the day and way sooner if it wasn't front-loaded correctly.

Dinner for Lunch

Vegetables rule. Where high-fiber grains, fruit, and dairy are important for breakfast, well-balanced, front-loaded vegetables are key to having a successful Big Meal of the Day that will fuel you until bedtime. The thing I love about the 7/7 Buffer Zone is that all or most of your just-in food (daily food intake) runs your waking hours and fat fuel keeps you going while you sleep. Add to your full-tank meal a nice mix of proteins (shooting for two fish servings a week) and you're in business.

67.2

Forty percent of 168 hours in a week is 67.2 hours. If we divide 67.2 by seven days in the week we get 9.6 hours. To pull off the 7/7 Buffer Zone you have to run your body on 9.6 hours or 9 hours and 36 minutes of fat fuel a day. To do that, we have to place 19.6 hours between our last meal of today and tomorrow's breakfast (10 hours of just-in fuel and 9.6 hours of fat burning). So that means we have a 4 hour and 24-minute window to get all of our nutrition in. A time to eat, a time to not eat. Less meals that mean more to us. If you've finished your dinner for lunch, let's say by one o'clock in the afternoon, then that would mean you couldn't have breakfast until 8:36 a.m. the next morning, 19.6 hours later. Like I said before, the 7/14, 7/11 Buffer Zones all work, too, and allow you to have more eating events a week but the 7/7 Buffer Zone is for that last bit of seemingly impossible-to-lose fat.

Life or Death

In a recent study, seven hundred adults with high blood pressure were assessed to see what difference their diet and eating times made to their health. The study focused on four areas: types of food eaten, amount of salt consumed, eating breakfast regularly, and the timing of evening meals. The research showed that eating dinner late had the most significant impact on your overnight blood pressure. People who had dinner within two hours of going to bed did more damage to their bodies than having a high-salt diet. Cardiologists at the world's largest heart conference concluded that the timing of our meals was critically important. They defined a healthy diet as having a good breakfast and lunch but limiting the last meal of the day to, at most, a light meal and to make sure that if you did have that extra light meal to consume it before seven o'clock.

Experts said that late-night eaters are more than twice as likely to die of a heart attack. Anytime we eat, it puts our bodies on "high alert," encouraging the production of stress hormones such as adrenaline. It's that adrenaline that keeps our blood pressure high and disrupts our circadian rhythms. While speaking at the European Society of Cardiology Congress in Rome, Dr. Ebru Özpelit, associate professor of cardiology at Dokuz Eylül University–Izmir, said, "Modern life was encouraging people into erratic eating habits which could cause damage over time." She went on to say, *"We must define the ideal frequency and timing of meals because how we eat may be as important as what we eat. Eating breakfast is important; we should have a strong breakfast and we shouldn't skip lunch."*

No more big dinners and no more eating after 7:00 p.m. was the message. The experts concluded what I figured out on my own: *The time between meals is as important as the meals themselves; and for our purposes, we call that space The Buffer Zone.*

Maintenance

According to CBS News, at any given moment there are 45 million Americans on a "diet." More than two-thirds of us are overweight or obese. And while losing weight may be our national pastime, keeping the weight off appears to be trickier than losing it in the first place. Sixty-five percent of us will gain back the weight we've lost and add a few pounds back within three years. That's a sad statistic. But I guess it makes sense; if so many of us try fad diets or quick weight-loss tricks, it's unrealistic to think we will have long-term success.

That's why the Buffer Zone is different. It's not a quick weight-loss or a fad diet; it is hard work. It trains your mind to flourish on fewer meals that are well designed so we can feel our best. The Buffer Zone is about adding nutrient-packed foods to our diet and blending them with the foods we know we love. If you love pizza and any diet says, "No more pizza for the rest of your life," you are destined to fail. Any food is only "good" or "bad" when it's compared to another food, but then it would just be one food is more nutritious than the other. Too much or too little of anything can be harmful.

Once I hit my desired weight and then kept dropping more weight, I bumped back up to the 7/11 Buffer Zone. Four days a week I have a primer breakfast, dinner for lunch, and a primer supper. Three days a week I have a primer-plus breakfast (40 percent of my caloric daily requirements) and then a full-tank dinner for lunch. Do I get cravings? Sure, especially when I'm stressed, but I always ask myself the one question that gets me out of it: "What's more important to me: what I want now or what I want most?" I might want a cookie now but I want to be healthy most. If I delay my cookie until I have my next full-tank meal, I'll literally get to have my cookie and my health, too.

Being healthy isn't about eliminating food I love from my life; it's about knowing there is a time and a place when I can have the food I love and there is a time and a place when I can't. I just remind myself what time it is. Self-control is a limited resource but fortunately we are always within twenty-four hours of getting what we want. For my entire adult life, I've been overweight, always fighting with one diet or another. The Buffer Zone saved my life. It can save yours, too. It isn't easy, but living with an overweight body isn't a walk in the park, either. I've been thin, I've been fat, and now I'm thin again. I prefer thin. I prefer healthy. It's hell to be fat, so I'm not going back there. Birthdays, anniversaries, and holidays will come and go. You will definitely see the scale move up when you indulge. But the good news is when it does, you know what to do. You buffer those pounds away.

I wish with my whole heart that life is good to you and that my little book makes a big impact. If it does, I've accomplished what I set out to do: make a difference in your life. We have one life, one body, one us. Let's take care of each other. I'll see you in the Buffer Zone.

All the best,
Fred

Epilogue

A t the end of chapter 8, I made a list of the things I knew, thought I knew, and knew I didn't know. Hindsight is 20/20. Let's go back to see what I got right, missed the mark on, and learned since then.

List 1: WHAT I KNOW

Of the twenty things I knew, I confirmed that seventeen out of the twenty statements were correct and discovered that statements one, eight, and nine need amendments.

1. *A lot of small meals each day doesn't help lose weight long term.*

    Not only do a lot of small meals (high frequency of eating events) not help with weight loss, it has the opposite effect: a high frequency of meals increases hunger and adds weight; lowering frequency reduces weight.

8. *If I skip a breakfast because I'm not hungry, I tend to be hungrier at lunch.*

One of the hardest things to do is to eat breakfast when you're not hungry. For example, when you're planning to have brunch on a Sunday morning, it can be tough to convince yourself to still eat a primer breakfast, as you don't want to spoil that delicious brunch. The problem is that when you don't jump-start your metabolism within the first two to four hours of waking up (2–4 Hour Rule) and the first meal of your day is a full-tank meal, it overwhelms your body. You end up eating too much at brunch (or any full-tank first meal) and when your body attempts to process that extremely heavy meal all at once, it can make you feel too full and put you in a "food coma."

Additionally, if you skip breakfast and merely have a primer for lunch, your body will attempt to play catch up and quickly expend all that new food energy within three hours. Although it isn't the end of the world to accidentally miss breakfast, skipping breakfast on purpose is a bad idea. Instead of spoiling a full-tank or primer lunch, small primer breakfasts start your engine and release any tension your body is holding on to by breaking your fast.

9. *If I eat a small, well-designed primer meal at lunch (even if I've skipped breakfast), I feel satisfied.*

Because of what I discovered in the previous statement, this is only partially correct. True, I felt satisfied, but the satisfaction didn't last. In my experience, if I skip breakfast and have a small primer lunch, the good energy I experience from eating takes a nosedive after only about three hours. In other words, it doesn't give me the five hours I need to get me to my next meal. Conversely, I realized that when I had a primer breakfast and a primer lunch, I could easily make it to my full-tank dinner.

List 2: WHAT I THOUGHT I KNEW

All twenty-one of the statements I thought I knew will now move to the "Things I Know" category because my research proved all of them are true.

List 3: WHAT I DIDN'T KNOW

This list identified forty-eight important things I didn't know. One could write entire books concerning each one of them. In an effort to learn about the things I didn't know, I took countless classes from the Teaching Company on nutrition and the human body. I would recommend anyone to do the same, as I now have a much deeper understanding of how our bodies work and how to take the best care of them.

Self-Discovery

In search of me
I fell victim to the stereotypes of others
I looked past the shores of circumstance
To find substance where truth and fiction
Change places at a whim

I reached out for answers
To questions that didn't exist
To find meaning in the ones that do
I evolved not out of chance nor fear
But to recognize my face in the mirror

My actions didn't always coincide
With the things that I believe
My convictions were occasionally afterthoughts
To the things that I achieved

But as my path outlined my direction
I find that I'm coming back home
My past becomes my present
My dreams no longer alone

As I reach beyond my grasp
I view an endless sea
I'm right back where I started
In search of me . . .

References

1. Allison, David B., and Monica L. Baskin. *Handbook of Assessment Methods for Eating Behaviors and Weight Related Problems: Measures, Theory, and Research.* Thousand Oaks, CA: Sage Publications, 1995. Print.

2. Appel, Lawrence J., et al. "A Clinical Trial of the Effects of Dietary Patterns on Blood Pressure." *New England Journal of Medicine* 336.16 (1997): 1117–124. *NEJM.* Web. 15 Feb. 2017.

3. Bellisle, France, Regina McDevitt, and Andrew M. Prentice. "Meal Frequency and Energy Balance." *British Journal of Nutrition* 77.S1 (1997): S57–70. *Cambridge.* Web. 7 Feb. 2017.

4. Burrows, T., S. Goldman, K. Pursey, and R. Lim. "Is There an Association between Dietary Intake and Academic Achievement: A Systematic Review." *Journal of Human Nutrition and Dietetics* (2016): n. pag. Wiley. Web. 7 Feb. 2017.

5. Chaix, Amandine, Amir Zarrinpar, Phuong Miu, and Satchidananda Panda. "Time-Restricted Feeding Is a Preventative and Therapeutic

Intervention against Diverse Nutritional Challenges." Cell. Elsevier Inc, 2 Dec. 2014. Web. 25 Jan. 2017.

6. Dixit, Vishwa, et al. "Controlled Meal Frequency without Caloric Restriction Alters Peripheral Blood Mononuclear Cell Cytokine Production." *Journal of Inflammation* 8.1 (2011): n. pag. *BioMed Central*. Web. 15 Feb. 2017.

7. Eckel, R. H., and R. M. Krauss. "American Heart Association Call to Action: Obesity as a Major Risk Factor for Coronary Heart Disease." *Circulation* 97.21 (1998): 2099–100. *AHA Journals*. Web. 31 Jan. 2017.

8. Fall, Tove, and Erik Ingelsson. "Genome-wide Association Studies of Obesity and Metabolic Syndrome." *Molecular and Cellular Endocrinology* 382.1 (2014): 740–57. *Science Direct*. Web. 6 Feb. 2017.

9. Flegal, Katherine M. "The Obesity Epidemic in Children and Adults: Current Evidence and Research Issues." *Medicine & Science in Sports & Exercise* 31.Supplement 1 (1999): S509–14. *Europe PMC*. Web. 31 Jan. 2017.

10. Frankl, Viktor E. *Man's Search for Meaning*. Boston: Beacon, 2006. Print.

11. Giskes, K., F. Van Lenthe, M. Avendano-Pabon, and J. Brug. "A Systematic Review of Environmental Factors and Obesogenic Dietary Intakes among Adults: Are We Getting Closer to Understanding Obesogenic Environments?" Obesity Reviews 12.5 (2010): E95–106. Wiley. Web. 7 Feb. 2017.

12. Giskes, Katrina, Gavin Turrell, Rebecca Bentley, and Anne Kavanagh. "Individual and Household-level Socioeconomic Position Is Associated with Harmful Alcohol Consumption Behaviours among Adults." *Australian and New Zealand Journal of Public Health* 35.3 (2011): 270–77. *Wiley Online*. Web. 7 Feb. 2017.

13. Giskes, K., G. Turrell, C. Patterson, and B. Newman. "Socioeconomic Differences among Australian Adults in Consumption of Fruit and

Vegetables and Intakes of Vitamins A, C and Folate." *Journal of Human Nutrition and Dietetics* 15.5 (2002): 375–85. *Wiley.* Web. 7 Feb. 2017.

14. Giskes, K., M. Avendano, J. Brug, and A. E. Kunst. "A Systematic Review of Studies on Socioeconomic Inequalities in Dietary Intakes Associated with Weight Gain and Overweight/Obesity Conducted among European Adults." *Obesity Reviews* 11.6 (2009): 413–29. *Wiley.* Web. 7 Feb. 2017.

15. Goldstein, D. J. "Beneficial Health Effects of Modest Weight Loss." *International Journal of Obesity and Related Metabolic Disorders: Journal of the International Association for the Study of Obesity* 16.6 (1992): 397–415. *Europe PMC.* Web. 6 Feb. 2017.

16. Gordon, Tavia. "Diabetes, Blood Lipids, and the Role of Obesity in Coronary Heart Disease Risk for Women." *Annals of Internal Medicine* 87.4 (1977): 393–79. *Europe PMC.* Web. 31 Jan. 2017.

17. Hart, D. J., I. Mootoosamy, D. V. Doyle, and T. D. Spector. "The Relationship between Osteoarthritis and Osteoporosis in the General Population: The Chingford Study." *Annals of the Rheumatic Diseases* 53.3 (1994): 158–62. *Europe PMC.* Web. 31 Jan. 2017.

18. Hatori, Megumi, et al. "Time-Restricted Feeding without Reducing Caloric Intake Prevents Metabolic Diseases in Mice Fed a High-Fat Diet." Science Direct. Elsevier Inc, 17 May 2012. Web. 25 Jan. 2017.

19. Hill, James O., and John C. Peters. "Environmental Contributions to the Obesity Epidemic." Science 280.5368 (1998): 1371–374. Science. Web. 6 Feb. 2017.

20. Hu, Frank B. *Obesity Epidemiology.* Oxford: Oxford UP, 2008. Print.

21. Jebb, Susan A., and Moore. "Contribution of a Sedentary Lifestyle and Inactivity to the Etiology of Overweight and Obesity: Current Evidence and Research Issues." *Medicine and Science in Sports and Exercise* 31.11 (1999): S534. *Europe PMC.* American College of Sports Medicine. Web. 31 Jan. 2017.

22. Kahleova, Hana et al. "Eating Two Larger Meals a Day (Breakfast and Lunch) Is More Effective than Six Smaller Meals in a Reduced-Energy Regimen for Patients with Type 2 Diabetes: A Randomised Crossover Study." *Diabetologia* 57.8 (2014): 1552–1560. *PMC*. Web. 25 Jan. 2017.

23. Kannel, William B., Naphtali Brand, John J. Skinner, Thomas R. Dawber, and Patricia M. McNamara. "The Relation of Adiposity to Blood Pressure and Development of Hypertension." *Annals of Internal Medicine* 67.1 (1967): 48. *Annals*. Web. 3 Feb. 2017.

24. Kondo, Marie, and Cathy Hirano. *The Life-Changing Magic of Tidying Up: The Japanese Art of Decluttering and Organizing*. Berkeley: Ten Speed, 2014. Print.

25. Kortt, Michael A., Paul C. Langley, and Emily R. Cox. "A Review of Cost-of-illness Studies on Obesity." *Clinical Therapeutics* 20.4 (1998): 772–79. *Science Direct*. Web. 7 Feb. 2017.

26. Ley, Ruth E. "Obesity and the Human Microbiome." *Current Opinion in Gastroenterology* 26.1 (2010): 5–11. *Lippincott Williams & Wilkins, Inc.* Web. 6 Feb. 2017.

27. Lissner, L., and B. L. Heitmann. "Dietary Fat and Obesity: Evidence from Epidemiology." *European Journal of Clinical Nutrition* 2.49 (1995): 79–90. *Europe PMC*. Department of Internal Medicine, Göteborg University, Sweden. Web. 26 Jan. 2017.

28. Lissner, Lauren. "Measuring Food Intake in Studies of Obesity." *Public Health Nutrition* 5.6a (2002): 889–92. *Cambridge*. Web. 7 Feb. 2017.

29. Luppino, Floriana S., et al. "Overweight, Obesity, and Depression." *Archives of General Psychiatry* 67.3 (2010): 220–29. *JAMA Network*. Web. 3 Feb. 2017.

30. Marks, Herbert H. "Influence of Obesity on Morbidity and Mortality." *Bulletin of the New York Academy of Medicine* 36.5 (1960): 296–312. Print.

31. Masuzaki, Hiroaki, et al. "A Transgenic Model of Visceral Obesity and the Metabolic Syndrome." *Science* 294.5549 (2001): 2166–70. *AAAS*. Web. 31 Jan. 2017.

32. Mejia, Michael. "Reach the Next Level: 5 Fresh Ways to Bust out of a Rut." *Men's Health*. Men's Health, 03 Aug. 2015. Web. 15 Feb. 2017.

33. Moro, Tatiana, et al. "Effects of Eight Weeks of Time-restricted Feeding (16/8) on Basal Metabolism, Maximal Strength, Body Composition, Inflammation, and Cardiovascular Risk Factors in Resistance-trained Males." *BioMed Central*. Journal of Translational Medicine, 13 Oct. 2016. Web. 25 Jan. 2017.

34. Obesity: Preventing and Managing the Global Epidemic. Vol. 894. Suiza: World Health Organization, 2000. Print.

35. Ovaskainen, M. L., et al. "Snacks as an Element of Energy Intake and Food Consumption." *European Journal of Clinical Nutrition* 60.4 (2005): 494–501. *U.S. National Library of Medicine*. Web. 7 Feb. 2017.

36. Pereira, Mark A., et al. "Dairy Consumption, Obesity, and the Insulin Resistance Syndrome in Young Adults." The JAMA Network. JAMA, 24 Apr. 2002. Web. 26 Jan. 2017.

37. Perrine, Stephen, Adam Bornstein, and Heather Hurlock. *The Men's Health Diet: 27 Days to Sculpted Abs, Maximum Muscle & Superhuman Sex!* New York: Rodale, 2013. Print.

38. Pi-Sunyer, F. Xavier. "Medical Hazards of Obesity." *Annals of Internal Medicine* 7th ser. 119.2 (1993): 655–60. *Annals*. Web. 6 Feb. 2017.

39. Reisin, Efrain, Franz G. Messerli, Hector O. Ventura, and Edward D. Frohlich. "Renal Haemodynamic Studies in Obesity Hypertension." *Journal of Hypertension* 5.4 (1987): n. pag. *Lippincott Williams & Wilkins, Inc.* Web. 7 Feb. 2017.

40. Rimm, E.B., et al. "Prospective Study of Alcohol Consumption and Risk of Coronary Disease in Men." The Lancet 2.8765 (1991): 464–68. The Lancet. Elsevier Ltd. Web. 25 Jan. 2017.

41. Ross, Amy. "Nutrition and Its Effects on Academic Performance: How Can Our Schools Improve?" (2010): n. pag. *Northern Michigan University*. Northern Michigan University, 28 July 2010. Web. 25 Jan. 2017.

42. Saunders, John B., Olaf G. Aasland, Thomas F. Barbor, Juan R. De La Fuente, and Marcus Grant. "Development of the Alcohol Use Disorders Identification Test (AUDIT): WHO Collaborative Project on Early Detection of Persons with Harmful Alcohol Consumption-II." Addiction 88.6 (1993): 791–804. Wiley Online Library. Society for the Study of Addiction. Web. 25 Jan. 2017.

43. Schmidt, Morten, et al."Obesity in Young Men, and Individual and Combined Risks of Type 2 Diabetes, Cardiovascular Morbidity and Death before 55 years of Age: A Danish 33-year Follow-up Study." *BMJ Open*. BMJ, 29 Apr. 2013. Web. 26 Jan. 2017.

44. St-Onge, Marie-Pierre, et al. "Meal Timing and Frequency: Implications for Cardiovascular Disease Prevention: A Scientific Statement From the American Heart Association." *Circulation*. American Heart Association Obesity Committee of the Council on Lifestyle and Cardiometabolic Health; Council on Cardiovascular Disease in the Young; Council on Clinical Cardiology; and Stroke Council, 30 Jan. 2017. Web. 31 Jan. 2017.

45. Summerbell, C. D., R. C. Moody, J. Shanks, M. J. Stock, and C. Geissler. "Sources of Energy from Meals versus Snacks in 220 People in Four Age Groups." *European Journal of Clinical Nutrition* 49.1 (1995): 33–41. *European Journal of Clinical Nutrition*. U.S. National Library of Medicine. Web. 07 Feb. 2017.

46. Szenas, P., and C. J. Pattee. "Studies Of Adrenocortical Function In Obesity." *The Journal of Clinical Endocrinology & Metabolism* 19.3 (1959): 344–50. *Oxford Academic*. Web. 7 Feb. 2017.

47. Tataranni, P. A., and A. Delparigi. "Functional Neuroimaging: A New Generation of Human Brain Studies in Obesity Research." *Obesity Reviews* 4.4 (2003): 229–38. *Wiley Online Library.* Web. 7 Feb. 2017.

48. Vollmer, William M., et al. "Effects of Diet and Sodium Intake on Blood Pressure: Subgroup Analysis of the DASH-Sodium Trial." *National Institutes of Health.* U.S. Department of Health and Human Services, 18 Dec. 2001. Web. 25 Jan. 2017.

49. Watson, Nathaniel F., et al. "Recommended Amount of Sleep for Pediatric Populations." Journal of Clinical Sleep Medicine 11.6 (2016): 591–92. American Academy of Sleep Medicine. The American Academy of Sleep Medicine and Sleep Research Society, 2015. Web. 25 Jan. 2017.

50. Wing, Rena R. "Physical Activity in the Treatment of the Adulthood Overweight and Obesity: Current Evidence and Research Issues." *Medicine & Science in Sports & Exercise* 31.Supplement 11 (1999): S547–52. *Europe PMC.* Web. 3 Feb. 2017.

About the Author

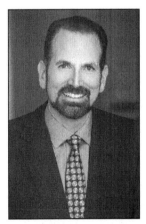

Fred Cuellar has distinguished himself in various fields. He is one of the world's top diamond experts, a three-time Guinness Book record holder in jewelry design, a consultant to investment and financial firms, and a best-selling author. His clients include the Dallas Cowboys, the Denver Broncos, the Detroit Redwings, plus celebrities associated with Lionsgate and the Rubik's Brand.

His personal commitment to making a difference in people's lives has taken him on a journey into the world of obesity, and his discoveries not only saved his life but can save yours.

Made in the USA
San Bernardino, CA
03 May 2017